AN AID TO
MEDICAL INTERVIEWS
AND
PROFESSIONAL DEVELOPMENT

An essential handbook for the junior doctor

DR. CHINMOY KUMAR MAITY
MBBS & MD (Calcutta); MRCP (London)
(Staff Physician; Department of Medicine; Leighton Hospital; Crewe
Formerly Specialist Registrar in Medicine, Charing Cross Hospital,
Hammersmith, London.)

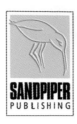

Sandpiper Publishing
Blackwater Lodge, Shop Lane
East Mersea, Colchester
Essex CO5 8TR

Tel: +44 (0) 1206 382271
Fax: +44 (0) 1206 382271
E Mail: salmonese@btinternet.com
www.sandpiperpublishing.com

Printed by
Healeys Printers Limited
Ipswich, Suffolk.

ISBN 0-9538606-4-7

*Dedicated to my known and unknown colleagues
across the globe who might benefit from this handbook*

Preface

The main reason behind my attempt in writing this handbook is the painful experience and difficulties I faced as a junior doctor at different levels of my career in getting information on the topics discussed here. The issues discussed in this book are very topical, quite useful in everyday practice and often questions are asked on these topics in interviews. There are a number of good books on each of these issues written by renowned authors in their respective fields. However, as a busy junior doctor or a clinician, we do not have the time to go through so much detail and practically we do not need them in great details in our day-to-day practice. The main purpose of this handbook is to give a brief but overall view on these topics to deal with them confidently in everyday practice. Nevertheless, for more detailed information on any particular topic, the reader is referred to relevant references given at the end of the book. Finally, my humble attempt will be considered as a success, only if the readers find it useful.

C K Maity

April 2004

Acknowledgements

In no way I am an expert in any of the fields or topics discussed in this handbook. Obviously I had to depend on different books and journal articles written by a number of authors, to whom I am indebted. I wish to acknowledge and express my gratitude to them. Many of my friends and colleagues have also supported me through constructive criticism, advice and help. I would like to mention here the names of two of my friends and colleagues – Mr. S N Ray, Specialist Registrar in Obstetrics and Gynaecology in Aberdeen and Dr. B H Willis, SHO in Medicine at Leighton, who himself is a statistician, for their invaluable advice and support in accomplishing my venture. Finally, I must thank my family for sparing me the time and space to complete this work.

Contents

Clinical governance

Background

The need for quality control measures in the NHS has been realised for a long time. The Bristol baby heart scandal (compared to other centres, a disproportionately large number of infants and children with congenital heart disease died after heart operations in the Bristol Cardio-Thoracic Centre and it was thought to be due to lack of necessary skills and competence of the concerned surgeons) in the late 1980s, however, shattered public confidence in NHS health care delivery. At the same time, it was revealed that the UK performs very poorly in international league tables of cancer death rates and more than half of all cancer patients are not being referred to an appropriate cancer specialist despite the Calman-Hine recommendations, which heightened public dissatisfaction further. The Department of Health (DoH) realised the urgent need for necessary steps to reform the NHS. The DoH, then, started publishing a series of documents
entitled **'White Paper'** issues.

NHS White Paper – Working for Patients (DoH, 1989) – addressed the issues of **clinical audit**.

The White Paper (DoH, 1997) – stated that the Government will require every NHS trust to embrace the concept of clinical governance centring around the issues of quality and accountability at organisational and individual level.

The First Class Service Quality in the NHS (DoH, 1998) – defined **clinical governance**.

Definition

"A framework through which NHS organisations are accountable for continuously improving the quality of their services and safeguarding high standards of care by creating an environment in which excellence in clinical care will flourish."

In other words, it is the involvement of clinicians and healthcare professionals to ensure quality and accountability in NHS healthcare delivery. The buzzwords are – Quality and Accountability.

Quality – is what outcome you want and being sure you get it, every time, for as long as you want it.

Accountability – is the responsibility of individuals or organisations for their action and the ability to explain and justify their activity.

Principles of CG

Principles of CG encompass a wide range of issues, of which the main ones are as follows:

1) Clinical audit.

2) Clinical effectiveness monitoring.

3) Clinical risk management – with adverse events being detected, openly investigated and lessons learnt.

4) Evidence-based practice.

5) Staff development – through lifelong learning and setting, maintaining and monitoring performance standard. Continuing medical education (CME), Continuing professional development (CPD), Record of in service training assessment (RITA), Appraisal and Revalidation are a few measures for the staff development.

Dimensions of CG

1) **Corporate accountability** – the accountable officer is the Chief Executive or the Chair of Governing Body of the NHS trust, who has the overall responsibility for clinical performance.

   A sub-committee led by a medical director or a chief nurse is responsible for the production of monthly reports of the trust board and a summary for inclusion in the annual report. NHS trusts produced their first clinical governance reports in Spring 2000.

2) **Internal mechanisms** – includes individual accountability, self and professional regulation, life-long learning, continuing medical education and continuing professional development.

3) **External mechanisms** – includes the following:

   a) **Commission for Health Improvement (CHI)** – is a statutory body which works like a watchdog. It provides national leadership to develop and disseminate clinical governance principles. It supports the NHS trusts to develop their local policies; visits the hospitals in regular intervals to assess the standard of care, find out any major defects in policy and helps to solve the problems.

   b) **National Institute of Clinical Excellence (NICE)** – is responsible for producing and disseminating clinical guidelines based on relevant evidence of clinical and cost effectiveness and associated clinical audit methodologies and information on good practice.

   c) **National Service Framework (NSF)** – develops protocols for management of various health related problems; eg. Coronary heart disease, Care of the Elderly etc.

   d) **National Performance Framework (NPF)** – is responsible for publishing local figures (eg. Death rates, complications rates etc.), to the public.

   Clinical governance is to play an important role in reorganising the NHS and restoring public confidence in NHS healthcare delivery. It has increasingly become an integral part of our day to day clinical practice.

Clinical audit

Definition

Audit is a quality control tool used to assess, evaluate and improve our practice by comparing with a set standard.

Medical audit is an integral part of our current medical practice. It is now compulsory for each and every NHS hospital to conduct monthly rolling half-day audit. In every NHS trust there is a defined Audit department, an Audit coordinator and a representative from each directorate to organise regular audits. All elective activities (Clinics, operations etc.) are cancelled during audit sessions.

Audit cycle

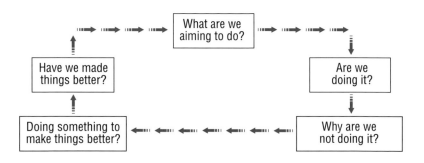

Steps in an audit

1) Select a topic and determine specific parameters to be studied.
2) Define your standards.
   a) <u>Gold standard</u> – national or international guidelines
   b) <u>Other standards</u> – local guidelines or accepted practice.
3) The Audit study – introduction / aims and objectives / methods / results / discussion & conclusion.
4) Highlight differences.
5) Recommendations / Develop coping strategies.
6) Repeat the audit study – 'closing the audit loop'.

Clinical effectiveness monitoring

Definition

Clinical effectiveness means 'doing the right thing, to the right people, at the right time and getting it right the first time'.

Measuring Clinical Effectiveness

Clinical effectiveness of any drug, intervention or policy is best assessed through randomised controlled trials. The NICE is responsible for assessing clinical effectiveness and producing guidelines for implementation in clinical practice. The stages of measuring clinical effectiveness are as follows:

- Ask the right question – which should be important, simple, specific, realistic, and focussed on an area where change is possible.
- Find the relevant evidence – by searching published literature, expert committee's opinion etc.
- Weigh up the evidence – as applicable in your particular situation.
- Apply the evidence in practice – by involving relevant peoples and over-coming barriers to application.
- Evaluate the changes – by making refinement to the application and continuing to monitor performance.
- Apply the evidence in wider context.

Monitoring Clinical Effectiveness

Continuing evaluation is necessary to monitor clinical effectiveness. The methods used for this purpose are – audit, assessment, appraisal and revalidation.

Clinical risk management

Definition

Clinical risk management is the process of detecting adverse events, investigating them openly and learning lessons from them to prevent further similar mishaps.

It is based on a framework designed to help identify the varied causes of **latent human failures** (inadequate organisational policies or inappropriate decisions – making the working environment more risky), **inadequate or inappropriate defences** (faulty monitoring equipments or procedures) and **active human failures** (making mistakes and breaking or violating rules or protocols).

Adverse incident & near misses

An **adverse event or incident** is defined as 'an unintended injury that was caused by medical management and that resulted in measurable disability'. In broader sense an adverse incident is 'any occurrence which is not consistent with the routine care of the patient or the routine operation of the institution'.

A **near miss** is defined as 'an occurrence, which but for luck or skilful management would in all probability have become an adverse incident'.

Hierarchy of risk management

The Chief Executive – has the ultimate accountability in the trust to implement the principles of Clinical Governance, of which clinical risk management is an important one. The final decision on a claim management is taken by the Chief Executive Officer, in consultation with the Medical Director, a non-executive director and the Director of Finance.

The Medical Director – is the chairman of the Risk Management Committee and the Incident and Claims Review Committee. In consultation with the Director of Nursing and the Risk Manager, the Medical Director implements policies to provide a systematic and strategic approach to the management of all clinical risks within the trust.

The Risk Manager – helps to design, implement and coordinate the Trust's clinical Risk Management Programme. He is responsible for implementation of hospital-wide risk education and prevention programme, induction programme in risk management for all new employees and development and maintenance of the adverse incident reporting system with agreement from the Risk Management Committee.

Risk indicators

A major component of the management of clinical risk is an agreed system for the reporting of clinically related patient incidents and near misses. One of the duties of the Risk Management Committee is to produce and review a list of **Risk Indicators**.

Some of the risk indicators are **non-specific** and some are specific **speciality based** (eg. surgical, obstetric, paediatric, anaesthetic, psychiatric etc). Examples of a few risk indicators are – misdiagnosis, medication error, failure to act upon abnormal pathology or imaging results, falls leading to severe injury or fracture, development of grade 3/4 pressure sores while on ward, surgery on wrong patient or wrong side, unplanned removal of an organ during surgery, neonatal or maternal death, delayed diagnosis of important congenital malformations etc.

An injured patient usually wants to understand the truth of what happened and to feel that steps have been taken to prevent recurrence. An honest explanation of the events and early apology, without necessarily admitting liability, often prevents future litigations.

Incident reporting & disciplinary action

Clinical risk management depends on effective and regular reporting of adverse incidents and near misses. Every effort must be made to avoid cover-ups of adverse incidents, mistakes and near misses. To implement an effective incident reporting system, the trust will have to establish a **no-blame culture**. The Chief Executive should ensure that no disciplinary action will result from reporting incidents, mistakes or near-misses, unless the behaviour is criminal, is malicious, constitutes gross misconduct or deviates from the trust's published policy.

The system of reporting adverse events must be simple, straightforward and understood by all staff. The use of a **single incident reporting form** will promote compliance. It is necessary to introduce an **explicit flow path** for the Incident Forms to ensure that incidents are all reviewed and graded by the Clinical Risk Manager before entry into the database and that the appropriate forms are then received by the Health and Safety, Occupational Health and other relevant departments.

Principal objectives

Clinical risk management aims to achieve four main objectives as follows:

- Early identification of latent failures and defence inadequacies, so that managers can act to remedy the situation before any accident occurs.

- Prompt incident reporting allows the Risk Manager to collect relevant records, necessary documents and witness statements relating to incidents soon after the accident, which helps defending the case to a great extent.

- Early warning of possible claims allows up-to-date evidence to be used by the trust to consider whether to settle or fight a possible claim or resolve a clinical complaint. Honesty with the patient and a move to an early equitable settlement (where appropriate) are usually better for the patient, the staff involved and the hospital.

- Early and structured investigation of the adverse incident helps to find the underlying failures or deficiencies and enables the hospital to learn lessons, so that safety can be enhanced and further accidents prevented.

Some other definitions

Clinical guidelines – is defined as 'systematically developed statements to help clinicians and clients in making decisions about care'.

Clinical protocol – is defined as 'locally adapted versions of the broad statements of good practice contained in national guidelines'.

Patient partnership – is the active participation of the patient and/or the patient's relatives in making decisions in the entire management plan.

Survey – means to have a general overview of a particular subject or matter. This is an observational study and there is no predetermined standard to compare with.

Evidence based medicine

Definition

It is a buzzword and there is a journal by the same title. Essentially, it means the conscientious and judicious use of the current and best available evidence from clinical research for management of individual patients.

The research-based evidence has to be used in the context of available clinical expertise and patients' preference.

Strength of evidence

Ia Evidence obtained from meta-analysis of randomised controlled trials.

Ib Evidence obtained from at least one randomised controlled trial.

IIa Evidence obtained from at least one well designed, controlled study without randomisation.

IIb Evidence obtained from at least one other type of well designed, quasi-experimental study.

III Evidence obtained from well designed, non-experimental, descriptive studies, such as comparative studies, correlation studies, and case studies.

IV Evidence obtained from expert committee reports or opinions and/or clinical experiences of respected authorities.

Grades of recommendations

A   Requires at least one randomised controlled trial as part of a body of literature of overall good quality and consistency addressing the specific recommendation (*Ia, Ib*).

B   Requires the availability of well controlled clinical studies but no randomised clinical trials on the topic of recommendation (*IIa, IIb, III*).

C   Requires evidence obtained from expert committee reports or opinions and/or clinical experiences of respected authorities (*IV*).

Implementing evidence into practice

Implementing research-based evidence into clinical practice may be difficult and time-consuming, as sometimes, it may require the health professionals to change their long-held beliefs and patterns of behaviour. The visible and measurable part of our professional practice is only the **tip of the iceberg**, which rests on the submerged broad base composed of our experiences, knowledge, values, attitudes, beliefs, assumptions and expectations. To get evidence into practice and bring about a change we have to:

- Consider individual beliefs, attitudes and knowledge likely to influence the behaviour of the concerned professionals and managers.
- Identify factors likely to influence the proposed changes.
- Plan appropriate interventions to overcome potential barriers.
- Be aware of the important influences in the organisational, economic and community environments.
- Motivate people to tackle the changes.
- Provide adequate resources.
- Incorporate monitoring and evaluation system from the beginning.
- Implement the change and find ways to maintain and reinforce the new practices.

Staff development

The fundamental aim of clinical governance is to provide a first class service with high standard of care to the patients. To provide a high standard of care the health care professionals should be well trained and up to date in their knowledge and skills, which in turn depends on continuing education and training and monitoring. One of the key objectives of implementation of clinical governance in the NHS is to establish the cultures of **learning, research and development** and encouraging **evaluation and feedback**.

The dynamics of provision of healthcare is based on three systems – **education and training, service** and **research and development**. The education and training system is designed, run and monitored by Post-Graduate Deanery and Education and Training Consortia in close co-operation with professional and statutory bodies like the Royal Colleges, Staff Training Committees (STCs), General Medical Council (GMC) etc.

The academic learning is provided via university-based system whereas the practical application of that academic learning is operated through the NHS Trusts and General Practices. The funding for education and training partly comes from the Health Authority allocations via three levies – Service Increment for Teaching (**SIFT**), Medical and Dental Education Levy (**MADEL**) and Non-Medical Education and Training Levy (**NMET**). SIFT is a levy which funds the additional costs to the NHS of supporting the clinical teaching of undergraduate medical students. MADEL covers part of the basic salaries of doctors in training and the local costs for the facilities for post-graduate medical and dental education like – maintenance of post-graduate centres and libraries, costs of study leave etc. NMET covers the costs of the education and training of professions other than doctors and dentists.

To keep up to date in knowledge and skills a professional will have to continue lifelong learning, ie. from cradle to grave of his / her professional career. This is called continuing medical education (CME) / continuing professional development (CPD).

A. CPD

Continuing professional development is defined as 'a process of lifelong learning for all individuals and teams which meets the needs of patients, and delivers the health outcomes and health priorities of the NHS and enables professionals to expand and fulfill their potential.'

This continuing education and training should be implemented at individual level, team level and organisational level and it should be multi-professional as well as uni-professional. CPD needs to be sensitive to individual and organisational needs. However, as these two needs are not always the same, there may be conflict between the service needs and professional aspirations.

The CPD measures at individual level includes – reading journals and textbooks, attending meetings, seminars and courses, presenting at meetings, research and publications.

Personal development planning is an important part of the CPD cycle. This includes a detailed set of **work objectives** and a detailed **training and development objectives**, linked to work objectives and both should be mutually agreed with individual's manager. They have to be supported by success criteria, deadlines for achieving the objectives and dates for reviewing progress in meeting those objectives.

All consultants and non-consultant career grade doctors are expected to maintain a **CPD diary** through **CPD Register** in their respective colleges (eg. RCP London).

B. RITA

Record of in service training assessment is a formal documentation of the regular assessment of the HO, SHO and Specialist Registrars in their training records. It is done by the educational supervisor and incorporates record of **core skills training**, **medical training**, **educational activities** and **appraisal**.

The trainees should have their first meeting with the educational supervisor during the first month of the post to set educational objectives for the period in which they will be working in the unit and to clarify their long-term aims. It is advisable that the educational supervisor meets the trainee informally midway in the post to check on progress. There will be a final assessment with appraisal at the end of the post.

RITA is the process of measuring or describing competence and performance against defined criteria based on relevant content. It is an opportunity to check progress regularly (usually annually) against the Core Curriculum. This is intended to provide support and guidance to trainees and trainers, and to assess the requirements of the post and whether the required standards are being achieved. It provides feedback from trainee to educational supervisor on the quality of the post and training programmes. Essentially RITA determines career progression and is entirely for the benefit of the trainee.

C. Appraisal

Appraisal is a process being introduced by the Department of Health for doctors working in the NHS. The aim is to give doctors regular feedback on past performance and continuing progress and to identify education and development needs for their career development.

Appraisal is – "A professional process of constructive dialogue in which the doctor being appraised has a formal structured opportunity to reflect on his / her work and consider how his / her effectiveness might be improved."

"A positive process to give someone feedback on their performance, to chart their continuing progress and to identify the development needs. It is a forward looking process, essential for the developmental and educational planning needs of an individual."

"The appraisal process is the vehicle through which the GMC revalidation requirements will be delivered. To this end appraisal discussions must be sufficiently broad to cover the essential requirements of revalidation."

It is the responsibility of the Chief Executive to ensure that Consultant's appraisal takes place regularly and annually.

Appraisers must be adequately trained in the process of appraisal. The Clinical Director is usually responsible for appraisal of consultants and non-consultant career grade doctors (NCCGs) in his/her directorate. The Clinical Director and if needed other consultants should be appraised by Directorate Lead Consultants or other trained appraiser appointed to an approved appraiser 'bank'.

Appraisal became a contractual requirement for consultants since 1 April 2001 and for GP principals since 1 April 2002. Appraisal for other groups of doctors, including non-consultant career grades, public health doctors, doctors in training and locum doctors will be introduced soon.

The appraisal process consists of discussion on the following issues:

1) Details of current job plan and activities.
2) Future personal development plan.
3) Good medical care (Evidence – current job plan/work programme, annual caseload/workload, list of audit work, etc).
4) Maintaining good medical practice (Evidence – up to date CPD certificate, certificate of attendance in national or international conference/meeting/ courses, etc).
5) Working relationship with colleagues (Evidence – 360° assessment report).
6) Relations with patients (Evidence – 360° assessment report).
7) Teaching and training (Evidence – feedback from teaching sessions (evaluation forms), letter from college tutor, etc).
8) Probity & Health (needs evidence if there is any problem).
9) Management activity.

Differences between appraisal & assessment

	Assessment	Appraisal
1)	Looks back	Looks back to look forward
2)	One way	Two way
3)	Pre-defined criteria / external standards	Discussion
4)	Pass / fail	Building
5)	Right / wrong	Improving

D. Revalidation

It is a process whereby doctors will have to demonstrate regularly to the GMC that they are fit to practise medicine. Doctors who are successful will be granted a licence to practise. Doctors who choose not to participate in the revalidation will be able to stay on the register without the entitlement to exercise the privileges currently associated with registration. If concerns are raised about a doctor's fitness to practise during the revalidation process, he / she will be referred to the GMC's fitness to practise procedures.

The revalidation process will be repeated every five years and it is mainly based on annual appraisal reports. First revalidation process for consultants is due to start in 2004.

Research

Definition

A systematic and rigorous investigation of materials undertaken to discover / establish facts or relationships and reach conclusions using scientifically sound methods.

It describes the processes and develops explanatory concepts ultimately to contribute to a scientific body of knowledge.

Why research?

a) To know 'what is the right thing to do?' and hence to practise evidence based medicine.

b) To become research literate (to read, write and understand papers).

c) To satisfy the requirement of academic career progression.

How is research related to audit & clinical governance?

a) **Clinical research** – answers 'What is the right thing to do?'

b) **Clinical audit** – answers 'Are we doing the thing right?'

c) **Clinical Governance** – ensures that the thing is being done right.

Types of research & study design

Research methods are primarily of two types, as follows:

a) **Quantitative research** – expresses mainly the investigators' viewpoint.

b) **Qualitative research** – expresses mainly the subjects' viewpoint. Qualitative research methods are particularly suitable for **primary care** research because of – i) their holistic approach, – ii) small numbers are acceptable and – iii) their focus on people as social being rather than as physiological systems.

Study design means a chosen method of collecting information necessary to answer a particular research question. Choosing a particular study design involves decision on:

a) Whether to intervene actively or simply describe what is observed **(Experimental vs Observational)**.

b) The timing for collecting information on exposure and outcome **(Prospective vs Retrospective or Longitudinal vs Cross-sectional)**.

c) The choice of control **(Parallel group vs Crossover study)**.

d) Randomisation **(Randomised vs Non-randomised)**.

e) Blinding **(Single blind or Double blind vs Open)**.

f) The **required sample size** etc.

A few common terms, used in various research study designs, are explained under the heading 'Research Glossary' below.

Research glossary

Experimental studies – the investigator can intervene actively and has some control over the study. So, the events are manipulated to some extent.

Observational studies – follow the natural course of events without any active intervention. These studies could be:

a) **Analytical** – where an exposure has been assigned (eg. Case control study, Cohort study and Cross-sectional study) or

b) **Descriptive** – where the natural course of events are observed and the outcome reported (eg. Survey).

Longitudinal studies – investigate a process over a period of time, which could be prospective or retrospective (eg. Cohort study, Case control studies etc).

Cross-sectional studies – observations are made at a single point of time. They are quick and cheap, but do not give any information about the causation or past of the disease (eg. Surveys, Prevalence studies etc).

Prospective studies – are also known as follow-up studies in which the data on exposure are collected first, and the subjects are followed up over a period of time for the development of a given condition or **outcome**. They give us valuable information on exposure, disease trend and impacts of the intervention in question. However, they need large sample, time and money.
Examples – Cohort study, Clinical trials etc.

Retrospective studies – are observational studies in which information on **outcome** (presence or absence of disease) is collected first, and the subjects are subsequently investigated for possible past **exposure** or a **risk factor** of interest.
Examples – Case control studies and rarely some Cohort studies.

Case control studies are usually retrospective studies, which start at the end point and go backwards in time to try to identify risk factors, which the subjects (known as **cases**) might have been exposed to in the past. The results are compared with a group of subjects without having the disease in question (known as **controls**, commonly selected through some form of **matching**). These studies are suitable for investigating rare diseases and needs relatively small sample size; however, they are very prone to **bias**.

Cohort studies – are prospective studies usually concerned with the **aetiology** of a disease or with the **prognosis** of those already suffering from a disease. They follow a group of individuals with particular risk factor, exposure or disease (known as cohort) over some period of time, until some **end point** (usually **death** or development of the **disease** of interest) is reached.

Crossover or Parallel group study – The commonest approach used in clinical trials is **Parallel design**, in which the new treatment is given to one group (the **treatment** or **test** group) and at the same time the conventional treatment or a placebo is given to a second group (the **control** group).

Crossover design – is a less frequently used approach in which one half of the subjects are given one treatment and the other half are given the second treatment. After a short washout period to prevent any carry-over effects, the two groups then swap treatments. As each subject in this study design acts as his / her own control, it needs a smaller sample size. However, it is not suitable for conditions which can be cured and high drop out rate is a common problem.

Controls – are subjects used in comparative studies to act as the standard against which new treatments or interventions are to be tested or the risk connected with a particular exposure, are evaluated. Controls can be concurrent or historical and they may be a different group of subjects or the same group as in crossover study.

Bias – is the systematic error which leads to results that are consistently wrong in one or other direction. When bias is present in an investigation, the validity of the results will be open to question. There are different types of biases:

a) **Selection bias** – randomisation is the best way to avoid it.

b) **Information biases** – are due to systematic errors in measuring **exposures** or **outcome**, which result in misclassification. They include Surveillance bias, Recall bias, Performance bias, Attrition bias etc.
Blinding is the way to minimise this bias.

c) **Confounding bias** – is the error, which occurs when groups being compared in a study are different with regard to important **risk** or **prognostic factors** other than the factor under investigation. In the **randomised controlled trials**, these confounding errors are minimised or avoided by making groups comparable in relation to known and unknown prognostic factors. However, confounding remains a main problem in **case-control studies**.

d) **Publication bias** – is the type of bias, which arises due to selective publication in medical journals of only those articles, which report **statistically significant** positive results. Given that the statistical significance is not synonymous with **quality, validity or clinical significance**, this practice can cause studies of poor quality and misleading results to have much greater impact on clinical and policy decisions than they merit. Also, good studies which have conclusively demonstrated a lack of treatment effect or lack of association (ie. a negative result) may never get to be published as their importance is often underestimated.
Systematic and **exhaustive review** of all published and unpublished studies on particular subject of interest is the way to avoid this bias.

Blinding – or masking is used in the context of **clinical trials**, whenever the participants (**single blind**) or both the participants and the researchers (**double blind**) are kept unaware of the treatment given or received. This avoids occurrence of observer and respondent biases (**information biases**). Placebos act as blinding measures in many trials.

Randomisation – is a process of allocating patients or participants to the alternative treatments or interventions in a **clinical trial**, with a view to produce comparable treatment groups in respect to important prognostic factors and thus, to minimise the **selection bias**. There are several methods of randomisation as follows:

a) **Simple randomisation** – the simplest way is to use a coin or a six-sided die or a table of random numbers (similar to using a ten-sided die). The main problem with this method is that it can not ensure that at the end of recruitment there will be equal number of patients in two groups.

b) **Blocked randomisation** – the allocation procedure is organised in such a way that equal number of cases are allocated to two groups. As an example, we can use a block of four containing two from each group in all possible combinations (eg. TCTC, TTCC, TCCT, CTCT, CCTT and CTTC).

c) **Stratified block randomisation** – here the confounding variables like patient's age, sex etc are taken into account to minimise selection bias further. Stratification can be made for any confounding variable, but it is usually advisable not to go beyond two variables. The method of balancing a large number of strata is known as **minimisation**.

Randomisation and blinding in a study allow all subjects to have equal opportunity to be assigned to either group and minimise bias and thereby assuring that any difference observed between the groups is purely due to by chance. Remote randomisation (telephone / internet) and double blinding are the best options.

Intention to treat analysis – in this study the patients are analysed in the groups to which they were randomised, ignoring the fact that some patients may drop out or be withdrawn from the trial. This approach minimises the bias arising from these situations.

Randomised controlled trial (RCT) – is the gold standard study design, but sometimes may not be feasible ethically. It has got the strength of having minimum bias, most precise estimation of effect and best quality evidence (Level 1), which can change clinical practice. The sample population is randomly assigned to experimental arm and control arm and the outcome of intervention is compared between the two.

The natural history of RCT involves:

1) Identify a research area / hypothesis.

2) Systematic review of literature.

3) Decide on the study population (Sample).

4) Decide on intervention.

5) Decide outcome measures.

6) Calculate the numbers required for statistical power.

7) Randomisation and Blinding.

8) Data collection.

9) Analysis of data by intention to treat.

10) Reporting of the trial results.

Non-randomised controlled trial (NRCT) – these types of trials are usually conducted in situations where randomisation is not possible, mainly due to ethical reasons. Usually a historical control is used in these types of studies. Examples:

a) Before-after (pre-test – post-test) studies.

b) Comparisons between matched groups.

c) Quasi-randomised trial – in which the treatment allocation is not random.

Meta-analysis – Statistical analysis, which combines the results of the individual studies used in a systematic review, producing a quantitative summary across the different studies. It uses methods like **Mantel-Haenszel estimates** and **Peto's method** to calculate these summaries. Meta-analysis has the virtue of increasing the sample size, but has the disadvantages of heterogeneity of samples and publication bias. Meta-analysis could be carried out on the original individual data from all studies involved or on aggregated data like odds ratios from each individual study.

Population, Sample, Data & Variables – all discussed under medical statistics.

Steps in writing a research proposal

1) Give a working project title.

2) Summarise the project.

3) Give the background of the study, with appropriate references.

4) Decide the aims (the overall goals of the project) and objectives (the specific tasks in stepwise sequence which will lead to the goal) of the study, or formulate a hypothesis.

5) Briefly describe the methods to be used, including design of the study, ethical considerations, data collection and analysis, interpretation of results, report writing and potential benefits to the NHS.

6) Describe the project milestones and devise a timetable to enable you to check that all stages will be covered and time allowed for writing up. In general, research time can be divided into thirds, one-third for planning and getting ready, one-third for data collection and one-third for analysis and writing up.

7) Generalisability, benefits to NHS and implementation of research findings.

8) Describe the likely costing for the project.

9) Apply for funding, if required.

10) Give references – use small number of references (fewer than ten), which should be accurate and well set out listing them in one of the standard styles, ie. **Harvard** or **Vancouver**. The later is the most popular style and involves numbering the references in the text, either in parentheses or superscripts, in the order in which they appear in the text. In Harvard style the name of the first author with the year of publication is cited in the text in parentheses and the reference list is written in alphabetical order.

Publications

Types of publications

1) Correspondence letter to the editor of a journal.

2) Writing a Case report.

3) Writing an abstract.

4) Writing a review article.

5) Writing an original article / paper.

6) Writing an editorial.

7) Writing a handbook / textbook.

Objectives of publishing a paper

1) Assessment of your observations by others.

2) Repeat the experiment if they wish.

3) To fulfil the requirement of academic career progression.

How to write a paper

Before embarking in to the expedition of research and publication, you must think about it carefully and never take it lightly. The important points to consider prior to the beginning of your new venture are:

- Is there any compelling need to do it? – It is really hard work.

- Do you have enough time? – It is time consuming. The time needed for your study can be divided into three equal parts – time for planning of the study and getting ready, time for collecting data and finally time for analysing data and writing up the paper.

- Have you got a predictable life-style? – You will need a stable personal, social and professional life and financial security to carry on.

- Do you have good library facility? – You will need it for your study.

Basic structure of a paper

Basic structure of a paper conventionally follows a format known as **'IMRAD'**, which is the abbreviation of Introduction, Methods, Results and Discussion. Nowadays, most journals print an **abstract** at the beginning of the paper and this is often the only part of the paper that people read. Each section of an article is meant for answering a particular question.

Abstract   What is, in brief, the main message from your study?

Introduction   Why did you start?

Methods   What did you do?

Results   What did you find?

Discussion   What does it mean?

a) **Abstract** – is a very brief summary of your study and it must contain the main points that you wish to get across. Every effort and sufficient time must be devoted to compose a good abstract and usually it should not exceed 250 words. Increasingly journals are now printing structured abstracts consisting of:
1) Objectives, 2) Design, 3) Setting, 4) Subjects, 5) Interventions, 6) Outcome measures, 7) Results and 8) Conclusion.

b) **Introduction** – should be brief and must state clearly the question that you tried to answer in your study. To lead the reader to this point it may be necessary to review the relevant literature briefly.

c) **Methods** – the main purpose of this section is to describe and sometimes descend the experimental design and to provide sufficient detail so that a competent worker can repeat the study.

d) **Results** – two key features of this section are – 1) overall description of the major findings of the study and 2) presentation of the data clearly and concisely.

e) **Discussion** – the total extent of discussion should not be more than the one-third of the entire article. It should include the following points:

1) Summarise major findings.

2) Discuss possible problems with the method used.

3) Compare your results with previous works.

4) Discuss the clinical and scientific implications of your findings.

5) Suggest a further work.

6) Present a succinct conclusion.

Final considerations

Once you have finished writing up your paper and the list of relevant **references** following one of the standard styles, you have to consider a few important issues before sending it for publication.

- Try to be your own sub-editor – you have to read your paper again and again to find out any mistakes, discrepancies, spelling and grammatical errors and make sure that the tables tally with your text.
- Choose a better word – you should always be in search for a better and more appropriate word in the relevant context.
- Try to give a short and catchy title.
- Find a particular journal - which might accept your paper for publication.
- You may have to change the style and format of your writing according to the requirement of a particular journal.
- If you have to send any photograph or radiology film, do not forget to label them on the back with authors' name, short title and indicate the 'TOP' with an arrow.

How to read a paper

'How to read a paper?' depends mainly on two important issues:

1) 'Why do you want to read the paper?' ie. the **purpose of your reading**.
2) 'Why was the study done or what clinical question the study tried to answer?' ie. the **purpose of the paper**.

Depending on the purpose, the reading can be classified into three types or levels as follows:

1) **Browsing** – means flicking through the books or journals looking for anything that might interest us.
2) **Reading for information** – in which we look through literature to find answer to a specific question or problem.
3) **Reading for research** – in which we have to go through the methodological details of the study and try to get a comprehensive view of the existing state of knowledge, ignorance and uncertainty in that particular field.

Critical evaluation of a paper includes assessment of – the appropriateness of the study, the methodological nitty-gritty, statistical significance, validity of the data presented, practical implications and cost-effectiveness. To enable us to this point we have to have the basic understandings about various **research study designs** and necessary **medical statistics**, which have been discussed in the preceding and the following chapters respectively.

Medical statistics

Basics

What is statistics?

__Statistics__ is a collection of procedures for describing and analysing data, whereas the data are the numbers we get when we measure and count things.

Types of statistics

1) __Descriptive Statistics__ – is used to describe the characteristics of a sample and it includes the followings:

   a) Methods for organising sample data.

   b) Methods for calculating average values.

   c) Methods for calculating values of spread.

   d) Methods of measuring association.

   Measures of average, measures of spread and measures of association of the sample values are collectively known as __summary measures__.

2) __Inferential Statistics__ – is used to draw conclusions from sample about the wider population from which the sample is drawn while taking into account the possible chance effects. It includes the followings:

   a) Confidence interval analysis.

   b) Hypothesis testing.

What is a variable?

A **Variable** is a name given to anything that can take on different values or attributes. Examples – age, sex, weight, height, blood groups, blood pressure, number of hospital admissions etc.

Types of variables – There are three types of variables as follows:

1) **Nominal or Categorical variables** – includes simple names or categories and they do not have any inherent orderings. Examples – yes / no, male / female, dead / alive, blood groups O / A / B / AB etc.

2) **Ordinal variables** – are the variables used to describe grades or stages and they have a natural or inherent ordering. Examples - grades or stages of a disease, degree of satisfaction (satisfied / undecided / unsatisfied), classes of heart failure or chest pain, level of improvement (much better / better / same / worse) or agreement (strongly agree/ agree / neutral / disagree / strongly disagree) etc.

3) **Metric or Numerical variables** – have precisely defined values and are real numbers which can be counted or measured. Examples – number of hospital admissions, age, height, weight, temperature, blood pressure etc.

We can apply all rules of arithmetic to metric data and they are also known as **Quantitative data / variables**.

Nominal and Ordinal data are not real numbers usually and we can not apply any rules of arithmetic to them; they rather express a quality and are also known as **Qualitative data / variables**.

Variables, which can take an unlimited number of values within a given range, are called **Continuous variables** and the data usually comes from **measuring** things. Examples - temperature, height, weight, volume, pressures etc, all of which are metric variables.

Variables, which can take a limited number of values or categories, are known as **Discrete variables** and the data usually comes from **counting** things. All nominal and ordinal variables are discrete. Some metric variables (eg. number of children per couple, number of birth / death / hospital admissions etc) are also discrete.

Discrete variables, which can take only two values (eg. yes / no, male / female, married / unmarried etc) are known as **Dichotomous variables** and the data is called **Binary data**.

Population & sample

A **Population** in statistics means a complete collection of a defined group of people, objects or items in which we have an interest. Examples – all school children in England, all drug addicts in London, all patients with stroke in a particular area, all prescriptions written last year from a GP Surgery etc.

A population includes every eligible member of the group however defined. Due to a number of reasons (eg. too large or too volatile population, limited resources, ethical and safety issues etc.), study of the whole population is impractical in most cases. To resolve this practical problem we draw a relatively small number of members from the population which is presumed to be a true representative of that population ie. that all the features of the population are accurately reflected in this small group called a **sample**.

Descriptive statistics

A. Organising data

After collecting the raw data, they are screened and listed into a number of categories with their respective frequencies in a table. A simple way to order and display data is to use a **Stem and leaf** plot.

Frequency distribution – A frequency distribution is a list of categories that a variable can take together with a count of the number of items in each category. When there are only a few categories (usually up to 15) they could be listed with one row for each category and it is called an ungrouped distribution. However, when there are many different categories they are grouped into a smaller and manageable number of classes for better understanding and analysis, which is called a grouped distribution.

Charting data – displaying data in the form of a chart often provides us more immediate impressionistic view and further insights into features and patterns in the data. There are a number of charts available for displaying different types of data as follows:

1) **For qualitative data:**

   a)   Bar charts   b)   Pie charts

   c)   Line charts   d)   Step charts (for cumulative frequency)

Bar charts are best used to display qualitative data with small number of categories and more than one variable can be plotted in the same chart. The bars are all of same width, equally spaced and the height of each bar represents the frequency of corresponding category. Example – distribution of patients with a particular diagnosis among seven consultants can be plotted as below.

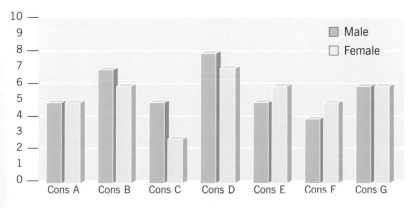

Pie chart is an alternative to bar chart, but it can display only one variable. The angle of each slice of the pie is proportional to the frequency of corresponding category and it is expressed in percentages. Example – the distribution of fifty consecutive asthma patients according to severity (mild, moderate or severe) can be displayed as below.

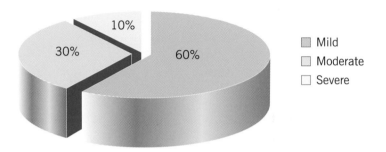

Line charts are used to display data with a chronological basis i.e. the data consist of regular measurements over a time period, which is known as longitudinal data. Example – number of daily admissions in a medical admission unit over a week can be plotted as follows:

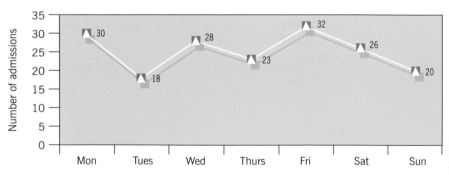

2) For discrete quantitative data:

a) Dot plots   **b)** Scatter plots

c) Frequency diagram   **d)** Step charts (for cumulative frequency)

Dot plot and Scatter plot are used to display ungrouped discrete data. Example – the relation between age and height in twenty children can be displayed in a scatter plot as follows.

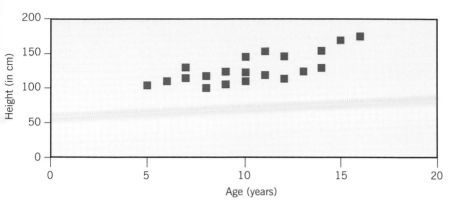

3) For continuous quantitative data:

a) Frequency histogram. **b)** Frequency polygon.

c) Frequency curve. **d)** Box-whisker plot.

Histograms are used to display continuous grouped frequency distributions. If the widths of the columns are same, the height of each column is equal to the corresponding class frequency. There is no gap between the bars/columns, which reflects the continuous nature of the data. Urinary lead concentration in a group of urban children is displayed in the following histogram.

If we connect the midpoints of all the columns of a histogram then we will get a curve, which is called a frequency polygon. A smooth frequency polygon is known as frequency curve.

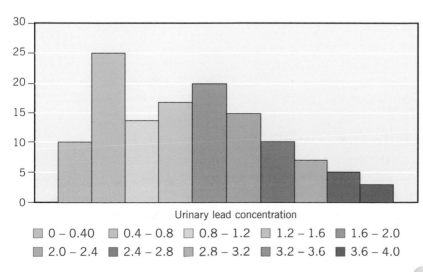

Frequency curve – the inherent patterns in the sample data are best understood by constructing charts. However, if the data are so distributed that we can draw a smooth curve through a frequency histogram or polygon then we get the ultimate realisation of this pattern and this curve is called a **frequency curve**. A frequency curve may be symmetrical or asymmetrical.

A frequency distribution, which has a smooth symmetric bell-shaped curve that can be described by a mathematical equation, is known as **normal distribution**.

An asymmetrical frequency curve having a longer tail on one side than the other, indicates a **skewed distribution**. When the frequency curve has a longer tail on the right side it is called **right** or **positively skewed** and similarly if the left tail is longer it is known as **left** or **negatively skewed**.

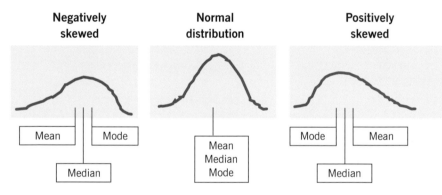

A frequency curve, which is flatter than Normal distribution is called **platokurtic** curve and one peakier than Normal distribution is known as **leptokurtic** curve.

Box-whisker plot is used to display a large data set. The bottom and top of the box mark the first and third quartiles. The horizontal line in the middle of the box marks the median and ends of the whiskers indicate the smallest and the largest sample values (ie. the range).

Box-whisker plot

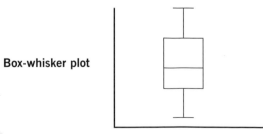

B. Measures of average or location

The commonly used measures are:

1) **Mean** – is the conventional average, which is calculated by adding up all the sample values and then dividing by the number of values.
   $\therefore \; \bar{x} - \Sigma x / n$. { $\bar{x}$ ('x bar') = mean; Σ (Greek capital sigma) = "sum of / summation"; x = each of the sample values; n = total number of sample values}.

2) **Median** – is the middle or central value after the sample values have been arranged in ascending order. If the sample values are even in number then the median is the average of the middle two values.

3) **Mode** – is the value that occurs most frequently in the sample data and measures the most typical value. A sample data having two modes is known to have a **bimodal distribution**.

4) **Percentiles** – are the values, which identify or locate any specified percentage of the whole sample. Examples - the values below which 10% or 25% of the sample values lie are known as 10th or 25th percentile respectively. The **50th percentile** divides the sample values into two equal halves and represents the median of the sample. The **25th, 50th** and **75th** percentiles are of particular interest as they divide the frequency distribution of the sample values into four equal parts and are known as first, second and third **quartiles**.

For metric data we can choose any of the measures of average from mean, median or mode and the choice depends mainly on which aspect of the average we wish to capture. For ordinal data mean should not be used and so the choice remains between median and mode. However, for nominal data the only suitable measure of average is mode. As a rule of the thumb the most appropriate measures of average are – **mean** for metric data, **median** for ordinal and skewed metric data and **mode** for nominal data.

If the frequency distribution is symmetrical then all three measures will be identical. If the frequency distribution is right or positively skewed then **mean > median > mode**; whereas in a left or negatively skewed distribution **mean < median < mode**.

C. Measures of spread or dispersion

Measures of spread or dispersion basically means the average distance of the sample values from the central value of the distribution. There are three types of spread measures:

1) **Frequency-based measures** – are based on the way in which the sample values are spread out among different categories or classes. They are principally used with nominal and non-numeric ordinal variables and include the – **variation ratio (VR), index of diversity (ID)** and **index of qualitative variation (IQV).**

2) **Range-based measures** – are based on the difference between the largest and the smallest values in the sample. They are used mainly with the numeric ordinal and skewed metric variables and include the – **range, interquartile range (IQR)** and **semi-interquartile range (SIQR).**

3) **Deviation-based measures** – are based on the average difference or deviation between each sample value and the mean of the sample values. They are used with metric variables and include – the **standard deviation**.

Standard deviation (SD)

Standard deviation (SD) – is the most important measure of spread used with metric variables. Steps in calculating standard deviation are:

Step 1: Calculate the sample mean value (**x**).

Step 2: Subtract this mean value from each observation (**X**) to get the **mean deviation** values (**X-x**).

Step 3: Square each of these mean deviation values (**X-x**)^2.

Step 4: Add these squared values together {Σ(**X-x**)^2}.

Step 5: Divide the sum by (**n-1**) ie. the degree of freedom. The result is known as **variance** {Σ(**X-x**)^2 / (**n-1**)}.

Step 6: Take the square-root of the variance and the result is the **standard deviation**. {**SD**=$\sqrt{\Sigma}$(**X-x**)^2 / (**n-1**)}.

When the sample values has a normal frequency distribution **68%** (68.27%) of sample values will lie within **one sd** of the mean and the corresponding figures within **two** and **three** *sd* of the mean are **95.45%** (95% within 1.96 *sd*) and **99.73%** (99% within 2.58 *sd*).

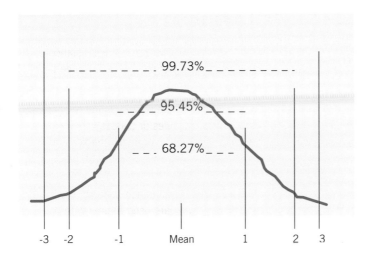

| -3 | -2 | -1 | Mean | 1 | 2 | 3 |

D. Measures of association

Correlation and regression

Correlation and regression are the techniques for dealing with the relationship or associations between two or more **continuous variables**. (χ^2 statistics is used for examining associations between discrete variables).

Correlation – denotes association between two quantitative variables and the degree of association is measured by a **correlation coefficient (r)**, which takes values between (+) 1 and (–) 1. Complete absence of correlation is represented by 0, whereas complete or perfect correlation between two variables are expressed either by (+) 1 or (–) 1.

A **positive correlation** is one in which both variables increase together. A **negative correlation** is one in which one variable decreases as the other increases. If change in one variable depends on change in another variable or the intention is to make inferences about one variable from the other, then the first variable is known as '**dependent variable**' and the other as '**independent variable**'. In graphical representation the dependent variable is usually plotted along the vertical axis or **y-axis** and the independent variable along the base line or **x-axis**.

Examples – (1) Association between age and height of a group of children, displayed in the scatter plot below reveals a positive correlation (*r = 1*). (2) Association between age and CD4 cell count displayed in the following scatter plot reveals a negative correlation (*r = -1*).

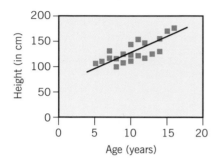

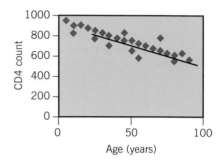

Correlation coefficient may be parametric **(Pearson's correlation coefficient)** or non-parametric **(Spearman's rank correlation coefficient)**. Parametric *r* quantify the extent of any linear increase or decrease; whereas, non-parametric *r* quantify the extent of any **tendency** for one variable to increase or decrease as the other increases.

The **Pearson's *r*** is calculated as: $r = \Sigma(X\text{-}x)(Y\text{-}y) / \sqrt{\{\Sigma(X\text{-}x)^2 (Y\text{-}y)^2\}}$, where

X represents the values of independent variable, **Y** represents the values of the dependent variable and **x** and **y** denotes the means of them respectively.

The **Spearman's** rank correlation coefficient (*rs*) is calculated as: $rs = 1 - \{6\Sigma d^2 / n(n^2\text{-}1)\}$, where *'d'* is the difference in ranks of the two variables for a given individual and *'n'* is the number of observations or categories.

The square of the correlation coefficient (*r²*) gives the proportions of the variation of one variable explained by the other.

The correlation coefficient is unaffected by the unit of measurement and it can not be used if the relationship is not linear. A significant correlation does not imply cause and effect (ie. correlation is not causation).

Regression - estimates the dependence of the dependent variable on the independent variable and the relationship is summarised by an equation known as **regression equation** consisting of a slope and an intercept. The regression equation is expressed as: $y = \alpha + \beta x$; where y is the dependent variable, x is the independent variable, α is the intercept representing the value of the dependent variable when the independent variable takes the value '0' and β is the slope representing the amount, the dependent variable increases with unit increase in the independent variable. The slope β is sometimes called as **regression coefficient**.

When there are more than one independent variables, the relationship is summarised by an equation known as **multiple regression equation** and is expressed as follows: $y = \alpha + \beta_1 x_1 + \beta_2 x_2 + \dots\dots + \beta_n x_n$; where x_1 is the first independent variable, x_2 is the second and so on up to the ***n*th** independent variable x_n.

Inferential statistics

A. Confidence Interval analysis

Standard error of mean (SEM or SE)

When we are studying a population we do not know the population mean (μ) or the standard deviation of the population mean (σ), we have only the mean of our sample to guide us. If we draw a series of samples from a large population and calculate the mean of the sample values in each of them, then we get a series of means. This series of means, like the series of observations in each sample, has a standard deviation. This standard deviation of the series of means is known as the **standard error of mean** of one sample. This standard error (SE) is a measure of how precisely the sample mean approximates the population mean. Repeated sampling from the population is a concept, but in fact we do not have to do that to calculate the standard error of the mean. It is calculated by dividing the SD by square-root of the number of observations (SEM = SD / $\sqrt{n}$). As with standard deviation, we can predict that a **sample mean** has a **95%** chance to lie within its two standard error from the **population mean**; in other words, a mean that departs by more than twice its standard error from the population mean would be expected by chance only in about **5%** of the samples.

Confidence Interval

It defines a range of values within which our true but unknown population mean value (μ) is likely to lie, with a given level of confidence. A single value or **point estimate** is likely to be inaccurate; but with this range of values (CI) we can be more confident (eg. 95%) that the population value lies within it. Conventionally we take 95% as the level of statistical significance and so, it is called 95% Confidence interval (**95% CI**). As the sample mean has a 95% chance to lie within its two standard error from the population mean, we can define **95% CI = $\mu \pm$ 1.96 SE**. However, we do not know the true value of μ. The best available data in hand about our pop-ulation is the sample mean, **x**. Conventionally, the best possible estimate of the confidence interval is measured using this sample mean. And so, **95% CI = x $\pm$ 1.96 SE**. Similarly we can calculate **90% CI = x $\pm$ 1.64 SE** and **99% CI = x $\pm$ 2.58 SE**. The narrower the range the more accurate is the estimate.

Standard error (**SE**) and Confidence interval (**CI**) analysis can be done on a number of parameters like **means, proportions, differences between means or proportions, regression coefficients, correlation coefficients and relative risks**.

The standard error of a **proportion** is calculated by the formula:
SE = $\sqrt{(pq / n)}$, where the **p** = proportion, the **q** = (**1-p**) and the **n** = sample size.

In case of means, the formula (**95% CI** = x $\pm$ **1.96 $\times$ SE**) applies for large samples. For smaller samples (roughly < 30), to get a reliable and accurate result, the **SE** of the estimate should be multiplied by the critical value of **t**, which can be found in the tables of the **t**-distribution against the appropriate number of degree of freedom (the **t**- test).

B. Hypothesis testing

When an investigator conducts a study he or she usually has a theory in mind; for example, patients with diabetes have high blood pressure, or oral contraceptives may cause breast cancer. This theory is known as the **study hypothesis**. However, it is impossible to prove most hypotheses; as one can always think of circumstances, which have not yet arisen, under which it may not hold. There is a simpler logical setting for disproving hypotheses than for proving them. The converse of the study hypothesis is known as the **null hypothesis**; eg. diabetic patients do not have high blood pressure or oral contraceptives do not cause breast cancer. Such a hypothesis is usually phrased in the negative and that is why it is termed **null**. **Hypothesis testing** is a method of deciding whether the data are consistent with the null hypothesis.

When we are studying the difference between two groups (eg. blood pressure in diabetic and non-diabetic patients or incidence of lung cancer in non-smokers and smokers) we must expect some difference due to **random variation** or **chance** alone.

We have to set a level of significance or limits before deciding whether the null hypothesis is true or false on the basis of the study results. The probability of obtaining an outcome as or more extreme than that observed in the study, if the null hypothesis is true, is known as the level of statistical significance or **P value**. Since the p value is a probability, it takes values between 0 and 1. Values near to zero suggest that the null hypothesis is unlikely to be true. The smaller the p value the more significant is the result. Conventionally we take 5% ($P = 0.05$) as the level of significance and we can get that by setting the limits at twice the standard error of the difference. So, a difference greater than the limits we have set is significant and makes null hypothesis unlikely. However, a difference within the set limits, which is regarded as non-significant does not make the null hypothesis likely, but it suggests that insufficient information is available to reject null hypothesis. $P = 0.05$ or 0.01 means the result is significant at 5% or 1% respectively; or in other words the sample difference has a 1 in 20 or 1 in 100 chance respectively of occurring if the null hypothesis is true.

Type 1 error – To reject the null hypothesis when in fact it is true is to make what is known as *type 1 error*. The level at which a result is declared significant is known as the *type 1 error rate* or α.

Type 2 error – The failure to reject the null hypothesis when in fact it is false is known as *type 2 error*. The *type 2 error rate* is denoted as β. The **power** of a study is defined as $(1-\beta)$ and is the probability of rejecting the null hypothesis when it is false. The probability of type 2 error or β becomes smaller with increasing sample size.

Null hypothesis

		False	True
Test result	**Significant**	Power	Type 1 error
	Non-significant	Type 2 error	Insufficient evidence.

Z-test & z-scores – 'z-test' is a significance test, which is used for comparing **means** or **proportions** between two groups. '**Z**-scores' are measurements, which are expressed in units of **standard deviation (SD)** or **standard error (SE)** and they are obtained by subtracting the mean from individual measurements (which follow a Normal distribution) and dividing the result by the standard deviation (SD).

So, **z-score** = (**observation** – **mean**) / **SD**. Example – if the mean height of a group of people is 170 cm with SD of 10 cm, a person measuring 180 cm has a z-score of 1 (ie. + 1 SD away from the mean).

Z-scores are used to assess the significance of a result by finding the appropriate P value in relation to the z-score from the 'P value table for a Normal distribution'.

The **higher the z-score**, the **smaller is the P value** ie. the result is unlikely to occur by chance.

Example – in a study, the mean difference in diastolic blood pressure between diabetics and non-diabetics was 6 mmHg and its standard error was 1.50 mmHg.

Now, we can assess whether this difference in BP of 6 mmHg is significant or has arisen by chance, by using z-score. Here the z-score is: 6 / 1.50 = 4, which means that this result is 4 SD away from the mean. From the 'P value table' we find that a SD of 3.291 represents a P value of 0.001. So, the above study result, being 4 SD away from the mean, has a P value of < 0.001 and is unlikely to be found by chance ie. the result is significant.

Significant tests

Statistical hypothesis tests are either parametric or non-parametric. The selection of an appropriate statistical test depends on:

a) Sample size.

b) Distribution of data.

c) Type of data (paired / unpaired or nominal / ordinal / metric).

If the sample size is large with an assumed Normal distribution in the population (however, lack of normality is of less concern if the sample size is large) and the data is metric, then calculation of the mean, SD, SEM and confidence interval are all that we need to assess the statistical significance of the study results. However, with small sample (usually < 30), skewed distribution, nominal / ordinal data the above tests will need some modifications to get reliable results.

1) **Parametric tests** – are used with the data assumed to have a Normal distribution, which could be characterised by a few parameters like the **mean** and **standard deviation**. Examples are:

   a) **_t_-test** (also called Student's t-test for the pseudonym "Student" used by the originator of t test, WS Gosset) which could be paired or unpaired.

   b) **z-test** – is used to calculate the z-score to determine the p-value, as described earlier.

   c) **Pearson's coefficient of linear correlation**.

2) **Non-parametric tests** – are used for the data which does not have a Normal distribution and so, can not be characterised by a few parameters, which is somewhat of a misnomer. These tests are also known as **rank score tests**, as they are usually based on rank. Examples are:

   a) **Wilcoxon test** – (conventionally for paired data).

   b) **Man-Whitney _U_ test** – (conventionally for unpaired data).

   c) **Spearman's Rank correlation**.

   d) **Chi-squared (χ^2) test** – this test can be carried out only on the actual number of occurrences, not on percentages, proportions, means of observations or other derived statistics.

   e) **McNemar's test** – is a special form of χ^2 test used in the analysis of paired proportions.

It can be argued that since non-parametric tests are distribution-free, they should be used always. However, the overwhelming arguments against the routine use of non-parametric tests are that they are not **flexible enough** and **less powerful** when used with data with a Normal distribution.

Choice of significant test

Choice of a suitable statistical test depends on a variety of factors, mainly the study hypothesis and the type of data (independent / paired, nominal / ordinal / metric).

While each case should be considered on its own merits, a rough guide in choosing a test is as follows:

a) For paired or matched observations

Variable	Test
Nominal	McNemar's test
Ordinal	Wilcoxon
Quantitative (discrete or non-Normal)	Wilcoxon
Quantitative (Normal)	Paired *t* test

b) For independent observations – choice of a statistical test is more complex and depends on input and output variables. A statistician's advice is recommended.

Sample size estimation

Sample size estimation is a crucial point in designing a trial for statistical power of the study. If the sample size is too small it will not be able to answer the question posed and the patients may be put at risk with no benefit but waste of time and money. On the other hand too large a sample will cause waste of resources where fewer patients would have sufficed.

The sample size for a **continuous outcome (unpaired data, measuring difference in means)** depends on four factors: the type 1 and type 2 error rate α and β, the variance of the data σ^2 (ie. SD^2) and the effect size d. The effect size, in a clinical trial, means the minimum difference that would be clinically worthwhile. The formula used to calculate the sample size per group is: $n = 2(Z\alpha+Z2\beta)^2\sigma^2 / d^2$ (Z = z-score). [The value of $(Z\alpha+Z2\beta)$ is easily available from a 'Table' to assist sample size calculation. Usually α and β are fixed at 5% and 20% respectively, setting a significance level at 5% and a study power $(1-\beta)$ at 80%. However, keeping $\alpha = 5\%$, the β can be fixed between 5 and 50%. For a β value of 20%, 10% and 5%, while α is fixed at 5%, the value of $(Z\alpha+Z2\beta)^2$ will be 7.849 (=**8**), 10.507 (=**10.50**) and 12.995 (=**13**) respectively.] Example – in a clinical trial in blood pressure reduction, if a clinically worthwhile effect for diastolic blood pressure is 5 mmHg and the between subject standard deviation is 10 mmHg, the required sample size $(n) = 2 \times 8 \times 10^2 / 5^2 = 64$ patients per group in the study.

The sample size for a **binary outcome (unpaired data, measuring difference in proportions)** depends on: α, β and proportions π_1 (the expected outcome under controlled intervention) and π_2 (the expected outcome in the control / placebo group). $\pi_1-\pi_2$ = the minimum clinical difference which is worthwhile detecting (d). The formula used is: $n = (Z\alpha+Z2\beta)^2 \{\pi_1(1-\pi_1) + \pi_2(1-\pi_2)\} / (\pi_1-\pi_2)^2$. Example – in a clinical trial suppose the placebo response is 0.25, and a worthwhile response to the drug is 0.50. The number of subjects required in each group so that we have an 80% power at 5% significance level is $n = 8\{0.5(1-0.5)+0.25(1-0.25)\} / (0.50-0.25)^2 = 55$.

In a **cross-over trial (paired data, measuring difference in means)** the formula used is: $n = (Z\alpha+Z2\beta)^2\sigma^2 / d^2$, where d = the anticipated difference between treatments and σ = standard deviation of the paired difference between treatments (not between subjects). Example – in a cross-over trial for arthritis, the within subject standard deviation of change in pain score (VAS) on getting out of bed from one period to the next is $\sigma = 3$ mm. If we wish to detect an improvement in pain scores between periods of 2 mm by use of a new drug with power 90% and significance level 5%, then the number of subjects required is $(n) = \mathbf{10.507} \times \mathbf{3^2} / \mathbf{2^2} = \mathbf{23.64} = \mathbf{24}$.

Diagnostic statistics

Diagnostic statistics plays a significant role in various diagnostic testing or screening tests and in our day-to-day practice of clinical medicine. A few commonly used terms in diagnostic statistics are:

Gold standard test – refers to a **valid** diagnostic tool, which consistently gives the correct diagnosis ie. **reliable** and **accurate**. In practice, gold standards are rarely 100% accurate, but they are simply the **best** method of diagnosis according to current dogma. Gold standard tests are often **invasive** or **expensive**, but can be used in studies to assess the performance (ie. sensitivity & specificity) of simpler and / or cheaper methods.

Incidence – of a disease is a measure of the number of **new cases** of the disease occurring during a specified period of time and is expressed with reference to the **person-time at risk** (eg. 5 per 1,000 persons per year).

Prevalence – of a disease is a measure of the total number of **existing cases** of the disease at a particular point in time (point prevalence) or a specified time period (period prevalence), divided by the total population or by the total population at mid-point of the specified interval. It is expressed per 100, 1,000 or 100,000 depending on the degree of prevalence. In the context of diagnostic testing prevalence is often used as an estimate of the **pre-test probability** of disease.

Probability – is the estimation of the likely prevalence of a condition or outcome of an intervention based on previous experience or educated guess. Probability is assessed by one of the three approaches – **frequency** approach, **model-based** approach and subjective approach.

Contingency tables (2x2) – are used to summarise the association between two categorical variables or binary variables. **Two columns** represent the different levels of one variable and the **two rows** represent the different levels of another variable.

This is a very important tool used to summarise data in **observational study**, **clinical trial** and **diagnostic testing**.

Example – In the context of **Diagnostic testing** this contingency table is used to calculate the following:

		Diseased		
		Yes	No	Total
	Positive	a	b	a+b
Test result	**Negative**	c	d	c+d
	Total	a+c	b+d	a+b+c+ d

Sensitivity – measures how good a test is in detecting those individuals who are truly diseased ie. detection of the **true positives**. ∴ Sensitivity = all testing positive and diseased / all diseased = **a / (a+c)**. The complement of sensitivity ie. (1-sensitivity) is the false negative rate **(FNR)** = 1-a / (a+c) = **c / (a+c)**.

Specificity – measures how good a test is in detecting those individuals who are not diseased ie. detection of the **true negatives**. ∴ Specificity = all testing negative and non-diseased / all non-diseased = **d / (b+d)**. The complement of specificity, ie. (1-specificity) is the false positive rate **(FPR)** = 1 – d / (b+d) = **b / (b+d)**.

Both sensitivity and specificity are not usually affected by the change in prevalence of the disease in question.

Positive Predictive value (PPV) – PPV of a test is the probability of actually having a condition given that the test result is positive. ∴ **PPV** = all testing positive and diseased / all testing positive = **a / (a+b)**.

Negative Predictive value (NPV) – NPV of a test is the probability of not having the condition given that the test result is negative. ∴ **NPV** = all testing negative and non-diseased / all testing negative = **d / (c+d)**.

Predictive values measure how useful a test is in practice and they are affected by changes in disease prevalence. A higher prevalence results in an increased PPV and a lower prevalence results in a decreased PPV. The opposite is true for the NPV.

Likelihood Ratio (LR) – The LR expresses the likelihood of finding the test result in patients with the condition relative to the likelihood of the same test result in patients without the condition.

∴ **(+) LR** = likelihood of +ve test result among diseased / likelihood of +ve test result among non-diseased = **{a / (a+c)} / {b / (b+d)}** = **_TPR / FPR.._**. A (+) LR>>1 is a good test for positive results ie. a positive result is more likely to be a true positive than a false positive.

∴ **(-) LR** = likelihood of – ve test result among diseased / likelihood of – ve test result among non-diseased = **{c / (a+c)} / {d / (b+d)}** = ___FNR / TNR___..
A (-) LR <<1 is a good test for negative results ie. a negative result is more likely to be a true negative than a false negative.

<u>Relative (Receiver) Operating Characteristics (ROC)</u> – when a diagnostic test produces a continuous measurement, then a convenient diagnostic cut-off must be selected to calculate the sensitivity and specificity of the test. For every possible cut-off value there will be a corresponding sensitivity and specificity. We can display these calculations by graphing the **sensitivity** (true positives) on the y-axis (vertical) and the false positive rate **(1-specificity)** on the x-axis (horizontal) for all possible cut-off values of the diagnostic test. The resulting curve is known as the **relative (receiver) operating characteristic curve** or **ROC curve**.

ROC curve demonstrates the trade off between sensitivity and specificity as threshold for test positivity is changed. A perfect diagnostic test would be one with no false positive or false negative results and would be represented by a line that starts at the origin and goes up the y-axis to a sensitivity of 1, and then across to a false positive rate of 0. A test with a **_TPR_ = _FPR_** would produce a ROC curve on the diagonal line y = x. Any reasonable diagnostic test should have a **_TPR>FPR_** and would display a ROC curve in the upper left triangle of the graph. Example:

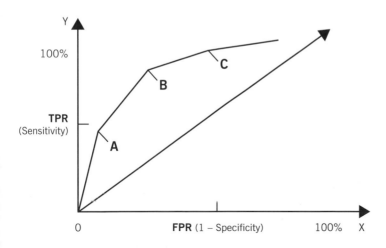

(**A** – high threshold for +ve; **C** – low threshold for +ve; **B** – is a reasonable compromise between sensitivity and specificity).

In the context of **Clinical trials** and **Observational studies** this contingency table is used to calculate the following:

		Exposure / Intervention		
		Yes	No	Total
Study outcome	**Positive**	a	b	a+b
	Negative	c	d	c+d
	Total	a+c	b+d	a+b+c+ d

Risk (R) & Risk Ratio or Relative Risk (RR) – means the probability of occurrence of an event within some given time period and these are used in **Prospective studies**. **Risk (R)** = number of events / number of people at risk = **(a+b) / (a+b+c+d)**. **Relative Risk (RR)** = risk in exposed group / risk in control group = **{a / (a+c)} / {b / b+d)}**.

Hazard Ratio (HR) – is the measure of **relative risk** used in **survival** studies. It is calculated as – $HR = (O_1/E_1) / (O_2/E_2)$; where O_1 and O_2 are the observed number of subjects with the event in groups 1 and 2 respectively; and E_1 and E_2 are the **expected** number of subjects with the event in groups 1 and 2 respectively. A HR of 1 means the hazard or risk of the event is the same in the two groups being compared. A HR less than 1 suggests group 1 is less likely to experience the event than group 2 and the opposite is true if the HR is greater than 1.

Odds & Odds Ratio (OR) – these terms are used in **Case control (retrospective) studies** instead of risk and relative risk respectively.

Odds = ratio of number of times an event occurs (P) to number of times it does not occur (1- P) = **P / (1-P)**.

Odds Ratio (OR) = odds in the exposed / odds in the non-exposed = **a / c : b / d = ad/bc**.

For rare diseases the OR and RR will be very similar. For a common event, for example a newborn baby being a boy or a girl, the probability or risk is roughly 0.5 or 50%, but the odds is 1 (50:50).

An OR = 1 means that there is no difference between two groups where as an OR < 1 is significant in favour of treatment or intervention.

Absolute Risk Difference or Reduction (ARD or ARR) – in comparative studies ARR expresses the benefit of one treatment or intervention compared with the other. It is also known as **attributable risk**. If the risk in study group is R_1 and the risk in the control group is R_2 then, **ARR = R_2-R_1 = b / (b+d)-a / (a+c)**.

Relative Risk Reduction (RRR) RRR is interproted as the proportion of the initial or baseline risk, which was eliminated by given treatment or intervention, or by avoidance of exposure or a risk factor. So, **RRR = (1-RR) x 100%**.

Number needed to treat (NNT) – it is a measure of the impact of a treatment or intervention. It states how many patients need to be treated with the treatment in question, in order to prevent an event, which would otherwise occur. So, **NNT = 1 / (R_2-R_1) = 1 / ARR**.

Bayes's theorem

Bayes's theorem was first introduced by Thomas Bayes. It explains a mathematical equation, which gives the conditional probability of an event, i.e. the probability that an event will occur given that another condition is also present. This is the basis for the calculation of the probability of disease given the results of relevant diagnostic tests. It includes:

a) **Predictive value of a test.**

b) **Multiplication rule.**

c) **Independence and mutually exclusive events.**

Essentially it allows us to revise our initial hypothesis on the level of disease in the light of further diagnostic information. We start with an initial hypothesis called a **prior** or **pre-test probability**. Then we apply the test, in which we know the characteristics. Based on the test information we modify our hypothesis to give a **posterior** or **post test probability**.

Steps in Bayesian analysis – Pre-test probability   Post-test probability

⬇   ⬆

Pre-test odds ➡ ➡ ➡ ➡ ➡ ➡ Post-test odds
Likelihood ratios

Pre test odds =   Pre-test probability / (1- Pre-test probability).
Post test odds =   Pre-test odds x Likelihood ratio.
Post test probability = Post-test odds / (1+ Post-test odds).

An example of Bayesian analysis (if conditional independence holds):

1) A man attends A&E with a history of chest pain. What is the probability of him having a MI?

- The prevalence of MI in those attending A&E with chest pain is 20%
- So, the **pre-test probability** of him having a MI = **0.20**
- The pre test odds = 0.20 / (1-0.20) = 0.25

2) Now, we know that he is **60 years old**. How is it going to modify the probability?

- The Likelihood ratio of having a MI in a 60 yr. old man with chest pain is = 1.8
- So, the post-test odds = 0.25x1.8 = 0.45
- The **post-test probability** of having a MI = 0.45 / (1+0.45) = 0.31

3) However, if the patient says that his **chest pain radiates to left arm**, but no **associated sweating**; how will it modify the probability?

- Chest pain radiating to left arm has a+ve LR for MI = 2.7
- Chest pain without sweating has a − ve LR for MI = 0.52
- So, the post-test odds = 0.25x1.8x2.7x0.52 = 0.63
- The post-test probability of having a MI = 0.63 / (1+0.63) = 0.39

Thus, a 60 years old man presenting with chest pain radiating to left arm but without associated sweating has a **39%** probability of having a MI.

Survival analysis

Survival analysis is concerned with studying the time between entry to a study and a subsequent event, originally concerned with death, hence the name. However, apart from mortality, survival analysis can be applicable to many other areas like − time taken to maximum exercise tolerance, time for a leg fracture to heal, time that a trans-dermal patch can be left in place etc.

When the outcome of a study is the time between one event and another, a number of problems can occur as follows:

- The times are more unlikely to be Normally distributed.
- We can not wait until the final events have happened to all the subjects and some patients may be lost to follow up. Thus the only information we have about some patients is that they were still alive at the last follow up. These are called **censored observations**.

If there is no censored observation, we may not necessarily have to use survival analysis; we can use a rank score test like Mann-Whitney U test. However, in survival analysis we analyse data using a **Kaplan-Meier survival curve** (a plot of cumulative survival probability against time).

Suppose that the survival times, including censored observations, after entry into the study of a group of **n** subjects are $t_1, t_2, \ldots, t_n$. The proportion of subjects, **S(t)**, surviving beyond any follow up time (**t_p**) is estimated by the following formula:

$$S(t) = \{(r_1-d_1) / r_1\} \times \{(r_2-d_2) / r_2\} \times \ldots \ldots \times \{(r_p-d_p) / r_p\},$$ when **t_p** is the largest survival time less than or equal to **t**; **r_i** is the number of subjects alive just before time **t_i** (the *i*th ordered survival time) and **d_i** denotes the number who died at time **t_i**, where **i** can be any value between 1 and p. For censored observations **d_i** = 0.

We can calculate the survival times **t_i**, for each value of **i** from 1 to **n**, by means of the recurrence formula: **$S(t_i) = \{(r_i-d_i) / r_i\}S(t_i-1)$**.

Comparison between two survival curves from two groups is done by **log rank test**. As multiple regressions is an extension of linear regression, the extension of log rank test in known as **Cox regression**.

Probability of survival of a group of patients with colorectal cancer, followed up over a period of seven years, is shown in following **Kaplan-Meier survival curve**.

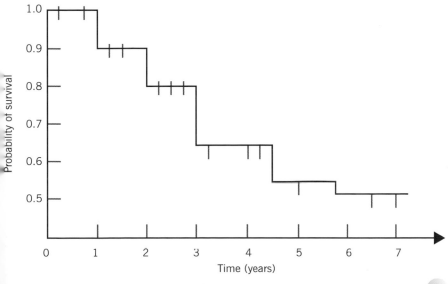

A few valuable tips for job interviews

Medical interviews are part and parcel of our professional life and we all have to face this one of the most nerve-racking experiences, when we move up the career ladder. Like in many other aspects of life, a certain amount of planning and preparation can make these experiences less daunting or even enjoyable.

Background

1) **How to write a standard Curriculum Vitae (CV)?** – the very first thing you have to consider before applying for a job is to write a standard CV. There is no hard and fast rule to follow any particular order or sequence in writing up the information.

   However, most hospitals have their own application forms for job application and they include most of the following necessary details.

   ● *Personal details* – which include your full name, correspondence address, sex, date of birth, marital status, nationality, GMC registration type and number (if you have one) and Medical Defence Union or Medical Protection Society membership number (if you have one) etc.

   ● *Professional qualifications* – you must list them in chronological order, putting the most current one first. You have to mention the years of qualifications and also the names of the Professional Bodies awarding the degrees.

   ● *Academic awards and distinctions* – you can list them even since your school level, again chronologically starting with the most recent one first.

   ● *Membership of learned societies* – include membership with learned societies like British Medical Association, Royal College of Physicians etc.

   ● *Present appointment* – it should include your grade, name and address of the department and hospital and the duration of your contract with the starting and finishing dates.

   ● *Previous appointments* – all previous appointments should be listed chronologically, starting with the most recent one first and it must include the details mentioned under present appointment.

- ***Clinical experience and skills*** – here you should mention briefly the experience and skills acquired from your previous jobs. You must mention your level of expertise in performing the practical procedures, those particularly required at your level. If you are applying for a Specialist Registrar post in some speciality, you can list the number of procedures you performed with and without supervision under a separate heading.

- ***Academic experience and skills*** – include your experience and skills in teaching, presentations, audits, research and publications. You should mention these under separate headings with brief description of your achievements in each field.

- ***Courses attended*** – list the relevant courses you attended in a chronological order and you can mention any particular expertise or skill you gained from them.

- ***Hobbies and interests*** – mention the main ones, especially one with some significant achievement and be ready to answer confidently, if you are asked any question on that topic.

- ***Career aspirations*** – here you should write your short and long term future career plans with a positive attitude.

- ***Referees*** – you have to give the names, addresses and contact tel phone and fax numbers of two to four referees, of whom at least one should be from your current job. You must ask permission from them beforehand for taking their names as referees.

2) **How to improve your CV?** – you must always try to improve your CV to increase your chance of being short-listed for the interview for your preferred post. The following few tips might help you in this respect.

- ***Attending courses*** – attending and having certificates of some courses like **ALERT** (Acute Life-threatening Events Recognition and Treatment), **BLS** (Basic Life Support), **ALS** (Advanced Life Support) and some speciality based courses (eg. Post Graduate Gastroenterology course, Endoscopy course, Echocardiography course etc) will improve your chance for being short-listed.

- ***Having additional/higher degrees*** – like BSc., Part 1 or full membership diploma or MD may be beneficial.

- ***Presentations*** – presentations in departmental journal club meetings, hospital grand rounds and especially in the regional, national or international meetings are very important.

- ***Participating in audit*** – is very important in this era of evidence-based medicine. You must participate in your departmental audits and be aware of your particular role played in the study.

- ***Research & publication*** – if you have one, that will definitely help you especially if that work is relevant to your next job. However, as a HO or SHO with a very busy work schedule and preparations for membership examination it is very difficult to have a research study or publication. To a great extent it depends on the interests of your supervising consultants. However, always be in search for a good/rare case for a possible **case report** and discuss your intention with your consultant.

Preparation

- Before attending the interview you must get a clear view of the post you applied for. You will get most of the relevant information from the job description and discussion with the person currently working in that post. It will be worthwhile to discuss about the post with the concerned consultant and even better to arrange a departmental visit, especially if it is a long-term rotation job or a permanent job.

- If you are attending interview for a new consultant post, you will need some special preparation. Attending one of the **Consultant Interview Courses** (eg. ***www.firstcourse-medical.co.uk***) will be very helpful. You must be fully aware of all the current health related **Government policies** (eg. revalidation, new consultant contracts, primary care trust, intermediate care, European Working Time Directive etc), **political issues** and **National Service Frameworks** (a good source for information is ***www.doh.gov.uk***). You should visit the hospital, discuss its current policies, future plans and any particular problems with the Chief Executive, Medical Director and relevant Clinical Director, colleagues and ward managers and read the annual report of the trust.

- Apart from some questions to judge your professional knowledge and competency in respective speciality, there are only a limited number of questions you can be asked in the interview. You should be aware of these common questions and prepare appropriate answers well in advance.

Presentation

While you present yourself before the interview panel, you must make sure that you look like a true professional. The following tips may help you in this regard.

- Plan your journey well in advance so that you can reach your interview centre much before your interview time.
- Dress yourself in conventional and sober dress.
- Try to keep yourself as calm as possible.
- Listen to the questions carefully and if needed, ask to repeat the question (not frequently).
- Try to avoid too much gesture.
- Keep eye contact with the interviewer and at times the other panel members while answering questions.
- Do not argue too much with the interviewer on any controversial topics.
- Do not forget to say '**thank you**' before leaving the interview room.
- If you have to give a **ten-minute presentation** on a particular topic to the interview panel, remember the following few points for a successful presentation.

a) ***Less is usually more*** – include a few essential key points to provide a clear and coherent coverage of a known topic. Avoid unnecessary details.

b) ***Keep each slide simple*** – five or six bullet-points a slide is usually sufficient. Each bullet-point needs to encapsulate a particular point, which you can explain in your speech.

c) ***Avoid high-tech tricks*** – try to keep your presentation simple, avoiding too much audio-visual effects. Always anticipate technical faults and be prepared to overcome it. Keep a back-up of paper copies and transparencies, which acts as a life-saver.

d) ***Watch where you stand*** – avoid turning your back to the audience. Whatever mode of presentation (computer or overhead) you use, always keep a paper copy at hand to avoid reading from the screen.

e) ***Keep to time*** – you must finish your talk within time, otherwise you will lose marks. Practising and timing your talk for a few times before the presentation will help you to get it right.

f) **_Question and answer time_** – you must prepare yourself well to answer the post-presentation questions stemming from your talk. You have to think about the possible questions and well-argued answers. You can discuss these with your colleagues for their views, which might be of great help.

A few common questions

The following common questions are asked in interviews to judge you as an individual professional, as a colleague team member and a colleague team leader and organiser. The interviewers do not have any interest in your personal details, which are irrelevant to the job. They are trying to select a colleague, who is honest, reliable, hardworking, flexible, knowledgeable and up to date in his field and level.

1) **_What makes you special? or tell us a little about yourself._**
This is a very common question to start with, in an interview. You should anticipate this type of question and prepare the answer. Do not reveal your personal details that are at best irrelevant to the job. Your answer should have a kind of past-present-future structure to link you and your past experiences to the job you are interviewed for. You can start with a brief background starting even before you went to medical school; then discuss your experiences gained in previous jobs including your key achievements, particularly those strongly related to your current interest and finally you should briefly tell your plan for future career development, in a way that suits the position you applied for.

2) **_What are your hobbies and interests?_**
With this question the interviewer is trying to find a little more about you, especially your energy and enthusiasm, morality, organisational skills and achievements outside your profession; ie. to see whether you have a healthy balance in your life. Participating in regular sports, organising on-call rotas, organising tours (expeditions, picnics etc.), doing voluntary work for charity and creative writing are some examples of good hobbies and interests, which are worth mentioning. If the interviewer has interest in some particular sports or current events, he / she might ask you a question on that topic; eg. 'What is your view about the performance of the England's cricket team in recent World cup series?'.

3) **_Tell us about your previous colleagues or consultants._**

The interviewer is again trying to unfold some other aspects of your character relevant to the job. Do not complain in any way about any of your previous colleagues or bosses, as this will never help you. However, you should not be too positive about your previous boss or job that is very different from the post you are now applying for. A reasonable way to answer this question is to describe how your previous job and colleagues assisted you in growing to become a better candidate than before. An account of any particular experience or achievement from your previous job is worth mentioning here.

4) **_If you could change one aspect of your personality, what would it be? or, what is your worst quality?_**

The answer to this question should focus on your self-awareness, your ability to take constructive criticism and feedback, and the ability to change yourself accordingly. Three types of bad qualities or weaknesses can be mentioned safely. Firstly, weaknesses those are entirely irrelevant to the job. Secondly, weaknesses that everybody has, as long as your one is not worse than others. Thirdly, the weaknesses you had in the past and been able to cure it with a positive attitude. Examples – you are very approachable and can not say 'no' to others; when you are busy and tired, you sometimes forget the need to take a short break and food and drinks; your habit to procrastinate a bit in the past before getting down to examine a patient, but you have corrected that since.

5) **_What is the worst mistake or failure you have had in your career?_**

When answering this question you must remember that this is an interview, not your confessional session and the art of winning this game lies in learning how to turn every question to your advantage. The best approach here is to admit to a mistake, which has absolutely no implications for the job itself or a weakness that everyone would admit to.

6) **_Why have you changed your mind about your career?_**

You must anticipate this question and prepare for a suitable answer if, you are going to attend an interview for a job in a speciality which is different from your previous speciality. Changes in career direction are common in medicine due to a variety of reasons. Do not feel embarrassed about your change in career direction; you should put forward the change as a 'development' rather than a 'mistake'. You must be confident to answer this question, but not defensive. Emphasise how much this new career path fits better with your strengths and interests than the previous direction you were taking. You should not forget to mention how incredibly the skills you acquired in your previous job, will be helpful in your new career direction.

7) _**Where do you see yourself in five years' time?**_

The main thing to remember here is that the interviewers want someone who is confident, ambitious and has an endless appetite for the kind of things they are interested in. The key to success in medicine is endless forward movement and the interviewers will not want someone who is going to be stagnant for five years. However, it is better to start humbly by saying that what happens in five years will depend on your performance in this job and the feedback you get. Make your long-term goal fit the job, but do not make the classic error of forcing the job to fit your deeper ambitions. Do not express any unrealistic expectation and do not aim to be somewhere further up the career ladder very much sooner than most previous incumbents have made it.

8) _**What are the duties and responsibilities of a good doctor?**_
**Or, If you are ill, what will you expect from your doctor?**

The answer to this question should be based on the General Medical Council's (GMC) handbook on '**Good Medical Practice**', which every GMC registered doctor is expected to read and follow. "Patients must be able to trust doctors with their lives and well-being. To justify that trust, we as a profession have a duty to maintain a good standard of practice and care and to show respect for human life without any discrimination." You must always be prepared to justify your action to them. In particular as a doctor you must:

- Make the care of your patient your first concern.
- Treat every patient politely and considerately.
- Respect patients' dignity and privacy.
- Listen to patients and respect their views.
- Give patients information in a way they can understand.
- Respect the rights of patients to be fully involved in decisions about their care.
- Keep your professional knowledge and skills up to date.
- Recognise the limits of your professional competence.
- Be honest and trustworthy.
- Respect and protect confidential information.
- Make sure that your personal beliefs do not prejudice patients' care.
- Act quickly to protect patients from risk if you have good reason to believe that you or a colleague may not be fit to practise.

- Avoid abusing your position as a doctor; and
- Work with colleagues in the ways that best serves patients' interests."

9) ***How can you organise a drug trial?***

You may expect this question or a similar question in the interview, especially if you have applied for a research post. The steps in organising a drug trial are as follows:

- Identify the need for a trial and arrange necessary funding – usually you have to find a Drug Company to sponsor the trial.

- Decide on the type of study design – whether it is retrospective or prospective; randomised or non-randomised; open / single blind or double blind; parallel group or cross-over trial and placebo or conventional drug vs new drug etc.

- Decide on inclusion and exclusion criteria – which is usually based on age, sex, racial and social factors and presence or absence of particular exposure, co-morbid conditions or concomitant use of other drugs etc.

- Define the end points (primary and secondary) – usually mortality or development of the disease in question or development of significant side-effects etc.

- Calculation of the power of the study – it is important to include enough number of patients to enable the trial to reach statistical significance and this is usually done with the help of a statistician.

- Ethics Committee approval – any trial should be approved by the Ethics Committee as per guidelines produced by the Helsinki Convention. The Ethics Committee requires detailed information as to the design of the trial and a consent form need to be approved by them.

- Decide on statistical tools for analysis – decide whether you need parametric or non-parametric statistical tests. The best approach is 'intention to treat analysis'.

- Interim analysis – it is important to analyse the end points as the trial proceeds, to detect any statistical difference should it become obvious at an early stage. Many trials have been stopped midway because a significant benefit or complication was so obvious that to continue the trial would have been unethical.

10) *How are you going to make a business plan for a new service you would like to launch in your department?*

This type of question is expected in an interview for a research post or a new consultant post. The intention behind the question is to judge your management and organising power.

When answering this question, you have to mention the **functions** of the proposed service, necessary **workforce**, **space** and **equipments** and a **budget proposal**. The steps in writing a business plan are as follows:

- Identify the need for a new service (a clinic or an investigation set up).
- Assess the extent of the need and the population to be served.
- Estimate the necessary resources and man power.
- Describe the likely costing for the initial set up and subsequent maintenance of the service.
- Suggest a possible source of funding, if applicable.
- Describe the project milestones in a stepwise sequence; and
- Mention the potential benefits to the trust.

11) *What do you think about the roles of specialist nurses?*

You can expect this question in an interview for a job in a speciality where specialist nurses play a significant role (eg. Specialist nurses in Diabetes, Heart failure, Asthma / COPD, Parkinson's Disease, Epilepsy, Urology, Stoma care etc).

They play a significant role in management of chronic medical / surgical problems which need longterm / lifelong care and supervision in the community as well as by the specialists in the hospital. They work as an important link between the patients in the community and the specialist doctors in hospitals and their role is beneficial for:

- Better continuity of patient's care.
- Better patient-professional relationship.
- Proven cost-effectiveness and
- Reducing the Specialist doctors' workload and waiting time in hospitals.

12) *How will you deal with one of your poorly performing colleagues?*

This is a very important question especially in a consultant's interview to assess your administrative quality and to explore a particular aspect of your character – your interpersonal relationship and your role as a colleague team leader. The interviewers are trying to find someone who is friendly, sympathetic and helpful to his colleagues, but at the same time is not ready to put the patient's safety at risk or compromise the standard of care.

An ideal answer to the question will be to deal with the issue in a stepwise manner and confidently as follows:

- To arrange a formal meeting with the concerned colleague in a friendly atmosphere to assess the situation and to explore any concern, worry, limitation or deficiency in his / her part.
- To advise him / her accordingly and to organise further training if indicated.
- To arrange a further meeting after a specified time period to reassess the situation and this may be included in the annual appraisal process.
- However, if he / she fails to improve even after several assessments or if his / her poor performance is serious enough to put patient's safety at risk or a criminal offence, then you have to bring it to the notice of your higher authority (eg. Clinical Director, Medical Director or the Chief Executive) for further action.

13) *How will you deal with a complaint? or* *How are the complaints dealt with in the NHS Trusts?*

In a democratic society we all have the right to complain against any public service authority and the NHS is no exception to that. A complaint can be made by a patient, patient's relatives or any NHS employee and complaints may be related to adverse events, malpractices or job related accidents.

The first point of contact in the complaints procedure in NHS Trusts is the **Patient Service Officer (PSO)**, who receives the complaint letter from the concerned party. The PSO then sends a copy of the complaint letter to the relevant clinician or manager for explanation. PSO usually arranges meeting with the concerned party to listen to them and explain the events in detail. The relevant clinician or the manager is usually present in this meeting to clarify the incident.

However, if the concerned party is not happy with the decision and actions taken, they may request for a review by the **Independent Review Panel**. Now the Trust's **Complaints Convenor** reviews the complaint and decides to refer the case either to an **Independent Expert's Review** or an Independent Review Panel. An Independent Review Panel consists of three responsible citizens, usually retired persons. However, depending on the nature of the complaint the panel may have expert members.

If the concerned party is still not happy with the decision even after the independent review, they may ask for a review by **Ombudsman** or go for litigation straightaway. Ombudsman is an official from an independent external agency appointed to investigate complaints against public authorities. If the Ombudsman's decision does not satisfy the concerned party, they may go for litigation.

Once the complaint is considered for a **Litigation**, it can be settled **out of court** with the agreement of both parties or may go to the **court** for a settlement.

So the pathway for a complaint management is as follows:

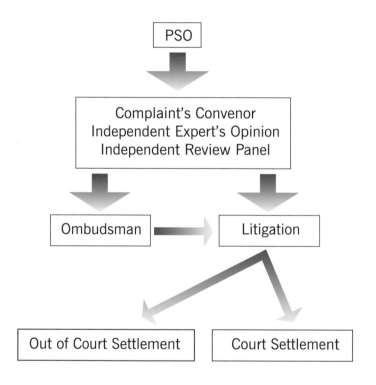

14) _Do you have any questions?_

This is usually the last question in an interview session. If everything went on very smoothly so far, you may finish by answering – 'No, I asked everything I needed to know already'. A better approach would be to ask a question which will reveal your interest in the post or the department. Examples – to enquire about the career progression of the predecessors or how the department is planning to cope with the new European working hours regulations etc. However, do not waste the interviewer's valuable time by asking a trivial question, which could have been answered by the hospital porter or the medical secretary organising the interviews.

15) ***Some other common questions.***

It is worth preparing some ready-made answers for them in advance.

- Why did you choose medical profession as your career?
- How do you know that you want to do medicine (or any other speciality you are giving interview for) for the rest of your career?
- If you are elected as the Health Minister of the country today, what major changes / improvements you would like to bring to the NHS?
- What are your strong points / weak points?
- Do you have any publication or presentation? If not, why?
- Have you participated in any audit? If yes, then what was your actual contribution in that study?
- Tell us about the duties and responsibilities in your current post.
- What do you specifically want to get from this job?
- If you get the job, what can the department / hospital expect from you?
- Are you prepared to take extra pressure and responsibility involved in the next step of your career ladder (ie. in the new job)?
- Can you tell us about a particular case that you managed very successfully and with great satisfaction?
- Tell us about a case that you did not manage well and learnt a lesson.
- Can you tell us about an interesting case, where you learnt a lot? / Can you tell us about an interesting case from your reflective diary? ('Reflective diaries' are usually maintained by the House Officers and medical students. An interesting case not necessarily means a rare / interesting medical problem. Management of a particular patient, which reveals your good communication skill, good interpersonal relationship and awareness of your own limitations, will be an ideal example to mention here).
- Have you worked in a multi-disciplinary team? / What is your view about the multi-disciplinary approach in patients' management?
- How are you going to break a bad news to the patient or patient's relatives?
- What makes you a good educator / researcher / clinician?
- What makes you tick (drive)?
- What non-medical book did you read lately?

- What are the NSF standards in your field / speciality (eg. Cardiology, Respiratory medicine, Geriatric Medicine etc)?
- How do you see your department / hospital in five years time?
- Why do you want to get a job in this particular region / hospital?

16) ***A few current issues*** *– which are very topical and important, especially for interview for a new consultant post, are discussed here briefly.*

i) European Working Time Directive (EWTD)

The Council of the European Union produced a directive to protect the health and safety of the workers in the European Union. It lays down the standard minimum requirements in relation to working hours, rest periods, annual leave and working arrangements for the night workers. This Directive was implemented in UK law as the **Working Time Regulations**, which took effect from 1 October 1998.

The key features of the EWTD are – an average of no more than 48 hours work per week, 11 hours continuous rest in 24 hours, 24 hours continuous rest in seven days (or 48 hours in 14 days), 20 minutes break in work periods of over 6 hours, four weeks annual leave and for the night workers an average of no more than eight hours work in 24 hours over the reference period.

The EWTD applied to all workers with a few exceptions, including doctors in training until now. From 1 August 2004 it will be extended to apply to the doctors in training as a legal requirement and also as a part of the wider aims to improve the work / life balance for NHS employees. However, the provisions will be phased in with a maximum hours requirement reducing from 58 hours in 2004 to 48 hours in 2009.

The British Government has applied a **'derogation'** which means that it is possible for a junior doctor to work more than 13 hours in a single shift, as long as those hours are not excessive and are compensated immediately to ensure a subsequent minimum of 11 hours rest period.

ii) Modernising Medical Careers – it is well appreciated that implementation of the EWTD will affect the work pattern of the doctors in training and will indeed challenge us to look at the way we deliver training. That is why the Government launched its Modernising Medical Careers strategy in February 2003 for a thorough review of the training systems and methods as well as looking at the end product of training.

In the mid 1990s the Chief Medical Officer (CMO), Sir Kenneth Calman, set the task of reorganising Postgraduate Education for junior doctors. He asked various colleges to produce a curriculum and after long discussion the Calman team produced the recommendations for each speciality, which is known as Calman Report. Calman reforms brought significant changes in the registrar grade training by amalgamating registrars and senior registrars into Specialist Registrars (SpR). However, the senior house officer (SHO) training has remained unchanged. This issue has been addressed by the present CMO, Sir Liam Donaldson, in his **Unfinished business**, which was sent out for consultation with the medical profession in August 2002. Following this consultation the Department of Health (DH) released document entitled *"Modernising Medical Careers"* which proposes the introduction of **Basic Medical Training (BMT)** programmes to replace the current SHO rotation programme.

It is **proposed** that the training period will be divided into three phases as follows:

1) **Foundation years (F1 & F2)** – The current pre-registration house officer (PRHO) year will be known as F1 and first year as an SHO will be known as F2. The F1 will include three or four-month modules rather than the traditional six months of medicine and six months of surgery. F2 is intended to give a broad base of training, with common learning goals which include acquisition of core skills and knowledge along with those outlined in the GMC document, **Good Medical Practice**.

2) **Basic Specialist Training years (BST)** – At some stage in F2 there will be competitive entry to one of the eight Basic Specialist Training programmes – Medicine, Surgery, Psychiatry, General Practice, Obstetrics & Gynaecology, Paediatrics and child health, Anaesthetics and Ophthalmology.

   In case of Medical programme, it is known as **Basic Medical Training** years 1 to 4 **(BMT1-4)**. BMT4 is the final year and is also considered as the first year of Higher Specialist Training (HST1). After satisfactory completion of BMT4 the trainees will be awarded a Certificate of Completion of Training in general internal medicine **(CCT-GIM)**.

3) **Higher Specialist Training years (HST)** – the duration and entry criteria to be set by each speciality.

In Medical programme, there will be an interview during BMT3 for entry into Higher Specialist Training. Depending on different sub-specialities the HST will continue between 2 to 4 years and after satisfactory completion of that period the trainee will be awarded a CCT in the Speciality.

The document "Modernising Medical Careers" also states that the non-consultant career grades (NCCGs) should be aided and facilitated to acquire a CCT. A Postgraduate Medical Education & Training Board (PMETB) has been formulated to organise competency based assess-ment. However, disappointingly there are no details as to how this might be achieved.

iii) **Improving Working Lives (IWL)** – is another initiative from the Department of Health and it sets out a series of performance standards for NHS employers to improve the working lives of the NHS employees. The aim is to encourage employers to develop a range of policies and practices which support personal and professional development and enable employees to achieve a healthy work-life balance. An IWL accreditation kite-mark will be awarded to the employers who can demonstrate, via portfolios of evidence, that they are improving the working lives of their employees.

There are three stages of development as follows:

1) *Pledge* – involves putting in place the people, policies and planning to achieve accreditation.

2) *Practice* – involves reaching the standard and putting policies into practice.

3) *Practice plus* – NHS employers achieving Practice accreditation will be reviewed by agreement between the Trust and their regional IWL accreditation team to check that any gaps in the standards have been remedied. Practice plus accreditation will be awarded when the regional IWL accreditation team is satisfied that the Standard is being met in full for all staff.

Targets to be achieved are as follows:

- *By April 2001* – All Trusts have achieved Stage One (Pledge) of the IWL accreditation.
- *By April 2003* – All NHS employers are expected to be accredited as putting the IWL Standard into practice.

iv) **Intermediate Care** – The Health system in UK is run until now by the

Local Health Authorities and it has a two-tier system – 1) Community based Primary care set up focussed on generalist approach and 2) Hospital based Secondary care focussed on specialist approach. The impetus for a new type of service called "Intermediate care" in the late 1990s was given a very considerable boost following the consultation on the National Bed Inquiry and the subsequent publication of the NHS Plan. An intermediate care type service will play an important role to bridge the gaps between the primary and secondary care.

The NHS Plan set out a major new programme to promote independence for the older people, through developing a range of services that are delivered in partnership between primary and secondary health care, local authority services, in particular social care, and the independent sector. One of the critical elements in this programme is to develop new intermediate care services. The NHS Plan announced an extra investment of £ 900 million annually by 2003 / 04 for intermediate care and related services to promote independence. The next target to achieve by March 2004 is at least 5,000 extra intermediate care beds and 220,000 people receiving intermediate care services.

Physicians have been somewhat ambivalent about intermediate care and the degree of involvement of doctors from primary and secondary care have been very variable in different parts of the country. Although intermediate care was conceived as an issue in all specialities, there has been very little secondary care input into intermediate care by other specialities apart from Geriatric medicine. Intermediate care is the **Standard three** in the **National Service Framework for Older People**. The aim of this standard is to provide integrated services to promote faster recovery from illness, prevent unnecessary acute hospital admissions, support timely discharge and maximise independent living.

Intermediate care has been seen as the solution to a number of different problems. From clinical viewpoint, it was seen as the reinvestment in rehabilitation type services, particularly for older people, in a properly organised multi-disciplinary environment, nearer to home, without the perceived dangers of prolonged in hospital care. From a managerial perspective, such services were seen as an answer to the chronic NHS bed crisis and to ensure that the NHS Plan targets for elective surgery could be met.

However, concern has been raised that development of intermediate care reflected an ageist policy being pursued by central government. The worry was that older people were being shunted into second rate under-resourced services and deprived of the resources and investigations available in district general hospitals. The intermediate care scheme should have build in clinical governance arrangements from their inception to protect against such discrimination.

A national evaluation of intermediate care has been commissioned and the result will be available in 2005/6.

v) **Primary Care Trusts (PCTs)** – In the late 1990s the British Government realised that the NHS was not fulfilling the people's expectation and that reform is the pre-condition for sustaining public confidence in the health service. It appreciated the public view that staff in public services have been simply doing their best inside a system that for too long has been under resourced and by and large people trust the NHS frontline staff (doctors, nurses and other health professionals). It also realised that most of the NHS frontline staff feel that the NHS is like a centrally run bureaucracy and the NHS can not be run from Whitehall.

With the above realisation the Department of Health launched the **NHS Modernisation Agency** and the **NHS Plan** to reform and redesign the NHS over a decade around the needs of the patients. This decade long modernisation process involves **significant structural reorganisation** and **huge cultural shift** in the NHS health care delivery. Department of Health planned to move the centre of gravity within the health service itself from **Whitehall** to the **NHS frontline** in a phased programme to decentralise the system and put power and resources in the hands of the NHS frontline. **"Shifting the Balance of Power"** within the NHS is the programme of change brought about to empower frontline staff and patients in the NHS and the main feature is giving the locally based primary care trusts the role of running the NHS and improving health in their areas.

The structural reorganisation plan involves – *a)* demolition of the existing 99 local health authorities and possibly all 8 regional offices and *b)* creation of new **Strategic Health Authorities (SHAs)** and transfer of extra powers to the **Primary Care Trusts (PCTs)**. The proposed boundaries of the new 28 SHAs were announced and they started functioning from April 2002. Each SHA covers an average population of 1.5 million and their main function is to support the **PCTs** and the **NHS Trusts** (secondary care trusts) in delivering the NHS Plan in their area. Although both NHS Trusts and PCTs will be accountable to the new SHAs, both will have greater operational freedom. NHS Trusts will be responsible for providing local hospital and specialist services. PCTs will be responsible for commissioning them as well as providing primary and community services.

The first 13 pioneering new Primary Care Trusts were announced by the Health Minister John Denham in January 2000 and they started functioning from 1 April 2000. Local GPs and nurses see and treat 90% of all patients seen by the NHS. They oversee how patients go into hospital, care for them when they leave hospital and work with social services and other agencies to look after them at home and in the community. So, the PCTs will be best run by these health care professionals who know the needs of their patients. PCTs will play a key role in developing fast, modern and convenient health services for patients. PCTs will give local doctors, nurses and other health professionals more control over the way the NHS develops than ever before. It will give them:

- A bigger say in how NHS money is spent than ever before. The typical PCT will control over 80% of the health spending on its local population.
- New power to provide local health services such as community nursing, community hospitals and service for the elderly.
- The power to work with the hospital clinicians to determine how other services are provided and to enable more services to be delivered closer to the patients.
- New powers to work with local health authorities to improve care of patients in the community.

All PCTs across the country are expected to start full functioning from 1 April 2004.

Further Reading:

1) **Clinical Governance** – Making it happen. Edited by Myriam Lugon & Jonathan Secker-Walker. Royal Society of Medicine Press Ltd. London & Illinois, 1999.

2) **Making Sense of Clinical Governance** – A workbook for NHS doctors, nurses and managers. Roy Lilley. Radcliffe Medical Press, Oxon, 1999.

3) **Understanding Research** – A scientific approach for health care professionals. Paul Stevens; Annette Schade; Barry Chalk & Oliver Slevin. Campion Press Ltd. Edinburgh, 1993.

4) **Research Methods in Primary Care** – Edited by Yvonne Carter & Cathryn Thomas Radcliffe Medical Press. Oxford & New York, 1997.

5) **How to do it** – Edited by Deborah Reece. BMJ Publishing Group. London, 3rd edition, 1995.

6) **How to Write a Paper** – Edited by George M Hall. BMJ Books, London, 2nd edition. 1998.

7) **CPD for UK Physicians** – The Federation of the Royal Colleges of Physicians of the UK. February, 2002

8) **Appraisal & Revalidation** – DoH & GMC join forces. GMC News; Issue 11, April, 2002.

9) **Consultant appraisal in the NHS** – Guidance for Appraisees and Appraisers. RCP - Education & Training. February, 2002.

10) **A Licence to Practise & Revalidation** – General Medical Council. April, 2003.

11) **Statistics from Scratch** – An Introduction for Health Care Professionals. David Bowers. Willey, Chichester, 1996.

12) **Statistics at Square One** – TDV Swinscow & MJ Campbell. BMJ Books, London, 10th edition, 2002.

13) **Statistics at Square Two** – M J Campbell. BMJ Books, London, 2001.